A Loving Voice II

A Loving Voice II

A Caregiver's Book of More Read-Aloud Stories for the Elderly

Edited by

Carolyn Banks
and
Janis Rizzo

The Charles Press, Publishers
Philadelphia

The Charles Press, Publishers
Post Office Box 15715
Philadelphia, PA 19103

Library of Congress Cataloging-in-Publication Data

A Loving Voice II: a caregiver's book of more read-aloud stories
for the elderly / edited by Carolyn Banks and Janis Rizzo.
     p. cm.
   ISBN 0-914783-70-X
   1. American literature. 2. Aged — Books and reading.
   3. Recitations. I. Banks, Carolyn. II. Rizzo, Janis.
   PS507.L622 /1994
   810.8'09285 — dc20   94-1593
                                       CIP
Printed in the United States of America
ISBN 0-914783-70-X
ISBN 13: 978-0-914783-70-1

Acknowledgments

"Some Games My Mother Played" © 1993 by Michael Dirda. An original story published by permission of the author.

"Picture Perfect" © 1993 by Lois Sargent. An original story published by permission of the author.

"Thelma's Quilt" © 1993 by Jean Adair. An original story published by permission of the author.

"The Open House" © 1984 by Christopher Woods. First published in *Story Time*. Reprinted by permission of the author.

iv

This book is dedicated to
Jon Reilman
and
Donald Banks
and to
Beth Whitley

Contents

Preface

When the first volume of *A Loving Voice* was first published, it received an enthusiastic and embracing welcome from the many different caregivers—those who were professional caregivers and family members and friends alike—who used the book. They were grateful to finally have at hand an anthology of suitable material that they could read aloud to the elderly people who were in their care. That there were no other books of this type—a book written deliberately for an elderly readership, not too simple, not too complex—undoubtedly contributed to the ongoing success of this book.

The appeal of this book to caregivers is straightforward: caregivers had learned—as indeed, Janis Rizzo and I learned when faced with the same situation in our personal lives—that no matter how much we loved those we were visiting in nursing homes, hospitals, hospices and at home, the time we spent with them all too often seemed awkward, a chore.

This isn't surprising. For one thing, what could we talk about to those whose capacities had diminished, whose world had grown painfully small and confined? It seemed cruel to talk to them about our own lives, our achievements, our travels. What was left to talk about?

We would do what we could. We'd bring in photos and old watches and articles of clothing in an attempt to court memories. We'd comb hair, rub backs, trim nails. And finally, we'd give up and turn on the television, hoping that whatever was flickering on the screen would in some way draw our loved one's attention. When the visit was up, we'd sigh with relief.

As I learned when working at an adult day care center, finding suitable reading material was not an easy task. Many activity directors who were reading aloud had actually resorted to reading children's books aloud to the elderly people they were trying to entertain. This troubled me. Though I recognize that there is a great deal of wonderful reading material for children, it seemed to me that this body of work excluded too much that older people had lived and known. It almost seemed patronizing, even though surely this was not intentional.

It was the realization of this need that made me conceive of compiling an anthology meant specifically to be read aloud to the elderly.

Janis and I began by soliciting stories and poems about adult experiences. We carefully edited those we selected so a listener would have no problem following the thread of a story, particularly with regard to dialogue.

We also looked for a variety of stories—suburban and rural, sad and glad. We included stories about young people, old people, pets and sports. Nothing, we decided, should be considered off limits. And we were extremely gratified when those who used the book wrote to tell us—and we received hundreds of responses—that we were on the right track; even enormously popular publications like *USA Today* praised the book.

We were thankful too when caregivers wrote to say they'd read all the stories and poems that were in the first volume of *A Loving Voice* over and over again and that they needed new material. Thus, we were encouraged to prepare the present second volume, *A Loving Voice II: A Caregiver's Book of More Read-Aloud Stories for the Elderly.*

As before, Janis and I hope that this book, like the first, will help you to find your own loving voice.

Carolyn Banks

A Loving Voice II

Some Games My Mother Played

by

Michael Dirda

My mother's father died when she was only two, leaving a widow and a dozen children to endure the Depression. Actually he left only eleven of his own offspring, but at some time my grandmother took in an abandoned baby who grew up to become one of my uncles. To this day I don't know which one.

It will probably seem like sentimental fiction to add that a railroad ran in back of my mother's childhood home and that she would help the family prepare for winter by picking up pieces of coal that had tumbled off passing coal-cars. Or that she first met my father as a little girl, stooping over a crayfish hole, waiting for a tug on her chicken-baited hook. Or that on summer evenings the neighborhood kids would play baseball in a nearby field, then scare each other with ghost stories as they ran from streetlight to streetlight on their way home. But so it was.

Years later my mother would tell her four mesmerized children about her childhood. No one could spin better stories, especially family histories or scary tales that would make her laugh with delight at our fear.

Once, when my father was working three to eleven, Mom

1

stood washing dishes; my sisters and I were playing or doing our homework. Suddenly, I heard a splash as a dish fell noisily into the water. I looked up to see our beloved mother unexpectedly drop to her knees, turn toward her children with a crazed look in her eyes, and start to make unearthly guttural noises. She growled and slavered, then began crawling toward us on all fours.

My sisters and I screamed, and ran with fast-beating hearts up to our bedroom where we locked the door. For a moment there was silence. Then we could hear the soft heavy sound of someone laboriously climbing the steps. On hands and knees. My sisters and I hid beneath our covers. Soon from outside the locked door came scratching sounds, and whimpers, as the Creature who had been our mother tried to get through to devour us. Then silence, followed by the noise of a hall cupboard being opened. We listened intently. Had It gone away? Suddenly we heard, with renewed hysteria, the jangle of a key being inserted into the lock, followed by our sanctuary's door slowly opening as the monster rushed into the room, laughing with insidious joy, scooping us into her arms and kissing us and telling us that she loved us and that we were all such suckers. Brazenly, we told her that we knew it was a joke all along.

My mother was never a sucker. In our family we children all learned to write our name, address and telephone number well before we started school. It was my mother's practice to take us with her grocery-shopping. Once arriving at the A&P she would deposit my sisters and me next to the store's raffle box. There, while she picked up bread and milk and looked for bargains, Sandy, Pam, Linda and I would fill out as many coupons as possible, as fast we could, dropping them into the foil-covered contest box, hoping to win turkeys or bags of groceries or money. And we did. Again and again.

My mother was serious about winning. We Dirdas always triumphed in coloring contests. After dinner, Mom would clear the table, set us down with the official Halloween or Christmas scene, and then tell us that we could only work on a single square inch for the next 15 minutes. It might take us two weeks to finish a pic-

2

ture, but when it was done, it was perfect. We won train sets, watches, dolls, cowboy guns, books, cameras.

Still, when it came to contests my mother was the undisputed champion. As my sisters grew up, she decided that each of them would need a sewing machine. Every year a local appliance store offered a contest, one in which people were challenged to make as many words as possible using any combination of letters from a long word like "disconsolate." The main prize was a portable sewing machine. Each year my mother would take out our family dictionary, and go through it, page by page, laboriously checking every single entry against the contest phrase. She took home the grand prize three years in a row, always generating hundreds more words than the runner-up. If she'd had more than three daughters she would certainly have kept winning sewing machines until each of her girls was provided for.

Still, my favorite memory of those early years concerns the new shopping center. In those days grand openings usually offered "Door-Buster" sales, with a handful of items marked down far below their normal selling price. When the Plaza opened near our house, my mom made sure we were all there, bright and early, at the front of the line. Like commandos, my sisters and I each had an assignment: when the doors flew open we would fan out across the store, hurriedly grabbing coats, skirts, jeans, what have you, before reporting back to our general, who would look over the merchandise and decide whether it would do for her family.

At this particular grand opening the shopping center also decided to hold a fair in its parking lot. On our way back to our car we passed a booth where people were throwing darts at balloons. Break a balloon and win a prize from one of the Plaza's new stores. I don't remember how much the darts cost, but my mother tried once, missed as most people did, and then packed up her kids and purchases and drove slowly home.

I thought no more about the matter, but my mother did. She found out that the same carnival would be coming through next May. That fall my mother bought a half a dozen darts and a target that she hung up on the door of the fruit cellar. For the next six months, whenever she was in the basement sorting or washing clothes, she would also practice with her darts. Upstairs we kids would hear the soft thonk, thonk, thonk as the darts hit the target. We were not allowed to play with them; they were like our father's tools—special and holy.

The next spring the Plaza held its May fair and my mother went over to the contest booth. She paid for her darts and proceeded to break balloons until they wouldn't let her play any longer. Typically, my mom didn't think it right that they should stop her from winning every prize in the place.

Picture Perfect

by

Lois Sargent

"What are you writing?" Howard asked his wife from behind his wall of newspaper.

"The Emancipation Proclamation," Sally shot back.

He nodded and proceeded from comics to business news with barely a rustle.

She put down her pen and closed her eyes in despair. When had the quiet reassurance in his eyes turned to bland sightlessness? Their romance had been the talk of the campus. Bubbly, outgoing Sally—Silly Sally they had called her—and good old reliable Howard. Her parents had been exuberant—whether over Howard or just relief that she hadn't run off with a troubadour, she wasn't sure. Their wedding had been beautiful. When she took Howard's arm she thought she had found her rock.

At first, when they were both working, things had gone well. They rented a small apartment and, after work, she always found so many things for them to do together. Howard would patiently go with her to flower shows, art galleries, estate sales. "My husband, Howard," she would say and he would smile his peaceable smile.

The good times might have gone on, too, but then they bought the house. It had seemed right at the time; everyone bought a house, settled down, and raised a family.

And so Sally quit her job and concentrated on the house and having children. Oh the love they lavished on the house!

She talked about having children; she talked about raising children; she talked about not concentrating so hard on having children.

She and Howard pursued hobbies. They took a course in photography together and they photographed the living, talking moments of their public and private lives. They filled an album with their photo-perfect lives.

Then they took up travel as a further distraction. They travelled on the weekends, on the holidays, during vacations. They photographed their travels.

She turned to writing. She had always wanted to write. There were so many things that she wanted to say. She wrote about her family, she wrote about her friends, she wrote about their travels.

And Sally rarely talked of children.

The house grew dowdy without love, so they stopped travelling and settled in. Routine began to build and mount into a siege against which Sally gave constant battle. While Howard was content, Sally developed dormant talents. She took charge of committees, she volunteered her time. Howard would smile at her conquests. He went to his job, performed his chores, and then engaged in confrontation with the daily newspaper.

And they rarely talked.

The years passed. So many years...

"Would you like some coffee?" she asked.

He raised his head rather quickly, "If you're fixing..."

Of course I'm fixing or I wouldn't have asked, she thought as she headed for the kitchen. The door swung shut behind her. She stood a moment savoring the darkness before turning on the cold fluorescent light—that remnant of a past decor. Howard had readily agreed that when she got published she could use her money to remodel the kitchen. She glowed at the thought of it. *Her* kitchen done *her* way with *her* money. His contribution to this

6

dream was smiling affirmation that rust and yellow would look better than this anemic green.

And she *would* get published. She knew it and felt it. Everyone in her writing class told her so. Mr. Jarvis always used her work as examples. This week she was scheduled to read. She could already feel the blush of pleasure the praise would bring.

Oh dear, the coffee pot was brimming over. She grabbed the towel draped on the oven door and with one whisk removed the boiling pot from the burner to the center of the stove.

Swoosh! The towel flamed along one edge. She hurled the burning towel into the sink and rushed to turn on the faucet.

Too late. Before she could reach across that porcelain abyss, the flames found friendship in the ruffled hanging of organdy about the window. Swoosh! The cold fluorescent light of the kitchen was brightened by a warmer glow.

"Howard! Howard!" she screamed. "Call the Fire Department! Quick!"

The flames were flickering along the cabinet walls. She watched, fascinated, as counter top items were consumed. She wanted to do something, but what? The flames blocked her from reaching the sink. She was vaguely aware of Howard's voice on the hall phone.

Swoosh! Another wall of brightness danced and teased before her eyes.

He startled her.

"Get out of here, Sally!" he urged as he tugged at her elbow. "There's nothing we can do. Get out! *Get out!*" he shouted as she stared, bewildered. He was pushing her back toward the door.

The flames danced and leapt frantically.

She turned and ran. She fled across the living room and down the hall. She found sanctuary in the bedroom. Her mind raced frantically. What to do? "Get out," Howard had said, but first...what to do?

Her eyes darted around the room. She hastened to the bureau, but found nothing there of consequence. She reached out toward the bed, resplendent with the intricate crochet produced by her own hands. Her fingers lingered on the spread for just a

7

moment before she directed herself to the closet. As her fingers glided past each garment, she shook her head in hopelessness.

She was aware now of the heat. "Get out!" he had shouted. Confused, she stared across the room until her glazed eyes focused upon their wedding picture on the night table.

She advanced toward the bureau, this time with a purpose. She extracted the album from the bottom drawer and with it safely in her arms, she fled the room.

The hall was smokey. And the flames! They were almost everywhere! She realized with terror that the fire was now stalking the living room.

"Howard!" she called. Where was he? She choked. "*Howard!*"

She could not reach the kitchen. She had to leave. He must have gone outside, she thought. "Get out!" he had said as he pushed her through the door. He must have returned to the den and gone out through the garage.

She was then out in the arms of neighbors. She inhaled deeply the fresh cool air. "Howard?" she desperately asked of them. "Have you seen Howard?" They gave comfort but no answer.

She clutched the album closely to her heart.

A small crowd had gathered. Most were familiar friendly faces, but they were disturbed now. She darted among the crowd. Howard was not with them. Sally dared to look back. She was astounded. The flames were reaching up and out. Where could he be? When she left him he was all right. He should have reached the door. He hadn't been frightened. He had been rough, determined to push her out and away.

"*Howard!*" she shouted hysterically. "*Are you out here?*" She dashed to the back of the house. Where could he have gone? There had been time to get out. She, after all, had gone back to the bedroom and still had time. He should have had plenty of time to get out.

"*Howard!*" she screamed again, nearly hoarse.

She was aware of sirens and knew help would arrive momentarily. She tightened her hold on the album. Her mind raced. *They'll find him. They'll get in and find him safely in some corner where he fell or got trapped or fainted. He probably made it to the den or the ga-*

8

rage; the flames haven't gotten there yet. She chewed her lip and a tear dropped onto the soft leather of the album.

How strange that this should happen to Howard—Howard who was always so careful, so organized, so correct in all his actions. What could have gone wrong? Safety had only been a door away. And he was going out the door behind her. He had pushed her. He had been behind her. He must have been. When she went down the hall, he must have gone out the door. She had been foolish to run to the bedroom. He hadn't followed her. She had been silly—Silly Sally—obsessed with saving something. She smiled half bitterly at what was now a bulky burden in her arms.

A shout from the crowd announced the arrival of the fire fighters. And then a more urgent shout came from the other direction. Sally couldn't quite make it out. Along the side of the house a man appeared, running, hunched over, giving protective custody to the contents he carried. "*Sally! Sally!*"

She ran toward him, weighted down by their albumed lives.

He was flushed from the heat of the fire. His face and hands were scratched; his clothing was disheveled and contained fragments of glass.

Howard was carrying a drawer, the center drawer of the desk. Howard smiled shyly at the sight of her and held out what he had salvaged. The drawer had been emptied of his ledger and bills. The usual receipts, all neatly stapled and categorized, were missing. If his well-maintained array of writing materials were still in there, they were hidden by a random clutter of her papers, her spiral notebooks, the envelopes in which she stuffed clippings and story ideas. And on top was her latest school assignment.

"I think," he said in his quiet way, "we'll need a future."

Thelma's Quilt

by

Jean Adair

When Thelma was a girl, she never touched a needle except to
sew an extra ruffle on her party frock. She hemmed no dishtowel,
cross-stitched no sampler, and as sure as the sun rises, she never
made a quilt. Oh, her mama sat her down a few times and made
her work on some nine-patch squares, but she only made four of
those. When Hiram proposed to Thelma, Thelma's mama and sisters made her a pile of quilts so she and Hiram wouldn't freeze in
their bed. (Thelma thought there was scant chance of that happening, but she didn't say so.)

Hiram and the children and the farm took up Thelma's
next thirty or so years. She learned to patch and hem. She sewed
aprons and rompers. One day, children grown up, housework
done, her bedding getting shabby, Thelma took a notion to make
a quilt. She got out her old nine-patch squares, sewed them together, and gave them a hard look. They were fine so far as they
went, but she didn't fancy making any more.

A red piece with yellow spots in the scrap bag took her eye.
It looked like the fat strawberries in her kitchen garden. Snip
with the scissors, bit of green wool for leaves, brown velvet for the
background. By late afternoon, a dozen strawberries had grown
in Thelma's hands. She sewed them all around the nine-patch.

Next day she rummaged in her scrap bag in earnest. She found calico as blue as the creek, sewed yellow fish to swim in it. She made Hiram's new Model-T out of shiny black satin. Outside, Thelma's apple trees foamed white and bore red. Inside, they blossomed and fruited on her quilt squares.

She made a square for each of her children and each of her sisters, one for Hiram, and another for Mama who had been called home long ago. She made her house and Mama's house with embroidered ivy swarming up the porch pillars. The Herefords, the sheep, the farm dogs, the barn cats, fat cabbages and skinny corn stalks all found their way into Thelma's quilt. At night red flannel tractors and pink cotton bachelor's buttons danced behind her eyes. By day they took shape in her hands, along with tomatoes in Mason jars, and onions and the windmill and the red-and-white striped tents at the county fair.

"Isn't that thing finished yet?" asked Hiram. "Looks pretty big to me." Thelma just smiled and stitched on. How could she put her life on a frame, stitch it together, hem it and call it done?

The crop blew away and the Depression blew in.

When the strawberries in the garden patch shriveled in the sun, the strawberries on the quilt patches gushed with juice. Hiram sold off the Herefords one by one—pitiful bony things they were toward the end—but they grazed perpetual gingham grass in Thelma's quilt, which by then was almost too heavy for her to lift.

One day the bank took the last sheep and Hiram watched the corn crop roast on the stalk. He came into the kitchen to sit and stare at his hands. Thelma went to the attic where she had stored her wool and began making a monstrous batting. She roused Hiram to drive two posts a good distance apart in the barnyard. She made him dig out four long timbers, left over from building the barn, and clamp them to the posts and to the hay wagon. She sewed together all the sheets she could spare and tacked this billowy tent to the timbers. With Hiram's help, she spread her batting on top and unfolded the quilt on that.

Then she cooked up a big stew of beef bones and the last of her canned vegetables, and sent for her neighbors and sisters.

11

The quilting bee went on for a week as there was scant chance of rain. The women sat on chairs in the barnyard and quilted and talked and quilted some more. Cars began stopping on the road, heads peering out of the windows. Planes overhead dipped their wings. A newspaper reporter came to ask dumb questions. ("They *would* send a man," Thelma grumped.)

Thelma didn't see her sister Betsy put the last stitch in the hem because Thelma was on her knees scrubbing the barn floor. She and the women and Hiram carried the quilt to the barn, where they tacked it to the topmost rafter of the haymow. It just cleared the floor as it fell in graceful folds across the empty stanchions. Thelma gave Hiram a piece of cardboard, a paintbrush, and instructions. Then she headed for the kitchen, where she began pressing apples. (The bank couldn't take the trees, after all.)

Thelma set the foamy pitcher of cider on an upturned crate in the yard along with her everyday tumblers and a cigar box for money. Hiram hammered the sign to a fence post just as the first of a parade of cars pulled in.

Even during the Depression, a nickel for a glass of fresh-pressed apple cider and another to see "The World's Biggest Quilt" was a bargain. People came from the 48 states and some countries that Thelma had to look up in her old geography book.

Over the years more reporters came, some from important magazines, some of whom were women for a change. "Is this really The World's Biggest Quilt?" they asked. Thelma's mama had taught her always to tell the truth, and she had her answer down pat, "I've never seen bigger."

"Do you consider yourself The World's Champion Quilter?" a reporter asked.

Thelma collected five more admissions and sent Hiram running for a fresh pitcher of cider. She cocked her head to admire the quilt hanging in the barn with the crowd of people gaping at it. Then she replied modestly, "No, not really. You see, I only ever made just the one."

12

The Open House

by

Christopher Woods

It was on a cold February morning that my father and I drove north on the interstate to the small town where he grew up. My father was born in that town, raised in a house his father had built. More than anything else, I knew this was a kind of memory trip for my father. His health was not good.

I had noticed how he had developed a habit of gazing into the past. It was a kind of looking-over-the-shoulder game that memory plays so well. But I also knew there was more space and time and dance of life in the past for someone whose future seemed as uncertain as his did.

We drove very slowly down Main Street in his old hometown. He seemed to study every sign and storefront, as if trying to memorize them. To me it was like a town gone elsewhere, without people, with a boarded-up drugstore and a long-closed five-and-dime. A theater sported a blank marquee, and a church seemed abandoned except for birds nesting in its eaves. It seemed that in that town, the people had gone, leaving only the physical things behind.

Stopping at a corner, my father pointed to a shuttered café where he and his friends once ate nickel hamburgers. It impressed me that he remembered the names of those friends,

13

though many years had since passed. I knew his memory was being coaxed, stirred by images of what seemed to me like a ghost-town childhood.

A surprise awaited us. When we arrived at his old address on Main Street where huge oaks buckled the sidewalk, where forlorn tree limbs pulsated in the cold air, there was nothing where his house had stood. Only a set of concrete steps announced what had once been a threshold. His house was gone. In its place was only a house open to the elements, a place that was a refuge of memory.

I knew memory could be like a piece of splintered wood, jagged and uneven. Or perhaps it was like a poem, only half-remembered. I knew that memory had to be summoned if it was to serve. It had to be awakened like sleepy monks for morning prayers. Memory sometimes needed to be pushed and shoved so that it could sing again.

This is exactly how it happened. Whether the house still stood or not did not bother my father. I followed him into his open house, myself recalling scenes from my own childhood played out there. He pointed to a place in the air where a frosted window had been, a milk-colored glass that glistened by day and became a glossy charcoal at night.

With his hands, he measured the length and width of the front porch swing, then the porch itself as it wrapped around the house, hugging it from every side. He showed me the woodshed, the scene of occasional whippings administered by his father.

I listened well, trying desperately to see his house as he still could, how it had stood, proud and high on stone blocks in the clearing between oak trees. The house was painted green and white, with tall gables. Listening, I began to understand that the real house no longer mattered. There are things passed down, one generation to the next. This house, his old home, was one of those things.

Maybe I didn't know many things, but I felt this was important. If waves and melodies and falling stars ceased to exist, they would all be lost unless they were part of a tale that is told again and again.

14

My father's house was no different. But there were some things he didn't have to tell me about. I knew them from my own life. The smell of summer in a dusty Southern town where shadows danced with heat. Or how June bugs shine and why they fear the dawn. Why in winter the icebound trees seem to have stars hung from every limb.

The frigid air bit at our skin as we headed back to the car. Later, on the way home, the heater turned on high, we spoke little. There was no need for words. The memory of his house had been passed down. It was complete; it was now a part of me.

I go easy on my memory when I am dredging it. It comes like some shrouded figure, a Lazarus emerging from a cave. Once I have coaxed it into the light, I study it to see what remains from before. Memory being a human thing, I am sometimes disappointed.

But sometimes I am pleased. Now, years later, my father's house is still there. It is as real as the wind that blows through its windows, to wake up the ghosts and send the lace curtains flying.

My Grandmother's Coat

by

Susan Volchok

I was there when she bought it. Of course, there was the usual hesitation, the mild but insistent anxiety about whether the coat was Too Good. As I recall, my mother stepped aside to let me handle the persuasion this one time. She shopped with my grandmother so often that some days, I suppose, she just couldn't muster the energy it took to argue Nanny Rose into being good to herself.

It wasn't that Nanny was the martyr-type some grandmothers choose to play. Self-aggrandizement, however disguised, just wasn't her style. She was far too modest to even *have* a style.

She never seemed to feel uncomfortable or deprived, never gave gloom and grimness any quarter, even when her life was at its hardest. It was as if she had no real concern for her own comfort and no realization of her entitlement to it.

Everyone else in the family should have only the best and she would make sure that we got it, if it were in her power. For herself, though, a butter-soft Italian purse (instead of a cracked vinyl satchel), a pretty velour wrapper (rather than a ratty terry), a pair of gold earrings, a bottle of imported perfume, were Too Good, at least for every day. So her drawers and closets were full of never-used things she was saving for Good Occasions, if such a hypothetical time should arise before she could get one of us to

16

take the stuff off her hands. Nanny's mania for giving it all away—nothing Too Good for her "kids"—was an endless source of family amusement.

And now, this coat: it was very, *very* good indeed, something special. My grandmother may not have instantly recognized the designer's name, but she knew a French signature in a coat meant it was out of her league. Still, patient as always, she played along at first as I persisted in buttoning her into the coat. A look in the mirror showed her what else the label meant—that it was a wonderful piece of work in navy wool, all crisp, clean lines and careful detailing, a chic coat that looked perfectly marvelous on her.

The coat was on sale—that's why we were there—and it was such a steal she had to agree it would have been a shame to leave it. As for its being too stylish, too elegant, Too Good for her, well, I just dismissed the idea as absurd, even teasing a shy smile out of her by telling her that I always wanted to see her looking as beautiful as she did in that smart blue coat. "Well…but this isn't a coat you wear every day," she demurred.

Dangerously close to losing my temper, I said shortly, "It's a coat I would wear every day." As if that were the best, most unassailable argument of all.

Did she ask me, then, whether I wanted the coat for myself? I seem to remember that she did. But I'm not certain if that's so, or if I only imagine it now because it was a question she was forever asking me: What did I want of hers? What could she give me?

I am certain that if she did ask, I answered "No!" impatiently, even rudely. I had never thought much about the real givingness that drove her queer desire to divest and do without. Nor did I realize that in finally agreeing to this coat instead of something plainer and cheaper, she was still giving. And not just giving in. She wanted to give me what I'd said I'd wanted—Nanny Rose in a new Trigère. From a certain point of view, she bought the coat as much for me as for herself, or perhaps more.

Predictably, she didn't don the coat that first season unless nagged into it. Too New always made Too Good even more intimidating. More than once, too, she urged me to take it. "You'll wear it," she said flatly. And when, annoyed, I demanded to know why

17

she couldn't wear it just as well, she shrugged, as if to imply some essential impediment, beyond mere words, to her strolling out of her little house in a handsomely tailored reefer instead of the worn storm-*schmatta* she stubbornly clung to. But, equally stubborn, I thought, *This is your new coat to wear and enjoy, for God's sake!* Why was such an idea so foreign to her?

It began to occur to me that perhaps this was something I couldn't do anything about. Eventually I contented myself with hoping the coat would age gracefully enough (as Nanny herself had) to remain a lovely thing by the time she finally reckoned it was ready for her—or she for it—say, four or five years hence.

Something else happened, though. The very next summer Nanny was feeling unwell for the first time in her eighty years. By autumn we knew that she was very sick, her lean and vigorous body concealing the cancer doctors predicted would kill her before summer came again.

When we took her to the surgeon's office, we bundled her into her big down coat for its reliable warmth and creature-comfort. It is true that Nanny's increasing frailness left her looking lost in the bulky embrace of the quilted down. But the designer wool would have presented a starker contrast still, as she shuffled along, her body bent, her belly hurting, her mind already closing, confused by what was happening and by the drugs and the pain that wouldn't stop.

After a while, when her rapid recovery from the stomach surgery-you could barely trace the scar-proved less than a miracle and Nanny relapsed into a slow, steady decline, she hardly ever went out at all. It was the middle of the winter then.

When spring arrived, Nanny remained in bed, too weak even to sit in the garden to which she had devoted many sunny days. She finally came to my mother's in early April. She didn't want to leave her house, but she couldn't take care of herself anymore. We packed a few things and wrapped her in her old storm coat for the short ride over. Her "new" French reefer stayed behind in the hall closet, smelling vaguely of camphor. We celebrated Mother's Day with her and then her eighty-first birthday, in May. She died in June, the day before summer.

When my mother felt up to it, she began to go through the possessions my grandmother hadn't managed to give away while she was alive—all she had left behind in the house where she'd lived with her dog and cat since my grandfather died almost fifteen years before. We were struck anew by the vast collection of untouched, Saved-for-Good things of every vintage, including—I had forgotten all about it by now—the coat. Did I want it? my mother was asking. *Déjà vu.* But my answer wasn't so fast, or so self-assured as before, when Nanny Rose had asked the same question.

On the one hand I so longed for my grandmother to be there, as she'd always been, that I coveted whatever pieces of her life I could possibly make my own. Yet, occasionally, I had the disquieting feeling of scavenging among her things as one might at some flea market. Moreover, it was one thing to treasure a ring or brooch she hadn't worn since her youth, or give a place of honor in my kitchen to her favorite pot or blade. But to shoulder my way into the coat I had willed her to choose for herself, the special coat that should by all rights have kept *her* warm for as many years as the one it had been intended to replace…. No, I didn't think so. As long as the coat was Nanny's, an end had not been reached. Not the absolute end. However dimly, I was aware that the emptiness of a coat eternally waiting on its wooden hanger was far more bearable than trying to fill that vacuum myself. That was beyond me at that time. It would have been too real a reminder of loss and distance.

Although the weather grew colder, my mother soon stopped asking me about the coat. She donated boxes of clothing to my grandmother's favorite Jewish relief agencies, but invariably, she left the coat out of each shipment. She couldn't, she said, give it away to "just anyone." For my part, I couldn't get it out of my thoughts. Sometimes I tried to imagine what it would really be like to slip on that elegant garment and step out of my own front door into the winter city. I took courage from the ease with which I could imagine Nanny Rose smiling to see me in a castoff coat so classy. I'd have to confess it was better than what I'd buy myself. It was even easier to imagine smiling back. Could I really refuse her offer?

I asked my mother to bring the coat along on her next visit.

This isn't the kind of thing you think your way through. The resolution came naturally, a small, almost unremarkable event. One twilight, after a long day working at my desk, I badly needed a walk in the park. And, needing a heavy coat against the wind that whips across the Hudson, I took my grandmother's out of the closet and buttoned it on in front of the hallway mirror. The coat fit as if it had been made for me. Slightly shorter than my customary length, it was all the more perfect for the jeans and sweaters it would top if I wore it…well, every day. I almost laughed out loud at the thought of this chichi thing serving as a sort of peacoat. Today—an ordinary day—felt as if it might be as good as life was going to get. Tomorrow everything could be changed, or gone. It was high time this coat got out on the town, even if that were only as far as Riverside Park.

In the park I headed up toward the community flower garden where I had sometimes gone to sit that summer, when it had recalled for me the wildly blossoming plants in Nanny Rose's yards. I slowly circled the garden, surveying the autumn ruins, and then turned back home. My hands were thrust into the silky depths of the coat's discreet pockets and I felt the weight and warmth of the wool against my body. I had turned the collar up and now I welcomed the semblance of privacy it provided: I was feeling sad suddenly, closer to tears than I'd been in a long time. Beneath the first rush of my resolve that the coat should be worn, and my unthinking pleasure in the sheer sensation of having it on, there was a sobering truth; my grandmother was far, far away from all this. Wearing her coat I realized—not for the first time, but with a fresh stab of certainty—how far away forever really is.

But as the darkness deepened around me and I climbed the path out of the park, my heart began to feel less heavy and my mind seemed to clear a little. The pain of absence still stabbed; I wished as I had never wished for anything that my Nanny Rose could be here walking with me under the trees in her own ever-new blue coat. And I knew what I was feeling wasn't the kind of sadness that one ever really gets over. But there was this: a glimmer, just a glimmer of gratitude that I had finally been able to accept her gift of the coat. For it seemed to me to signify some deeper acceptance, not just of her loss, but also of her love.

I've always mistrusted it when people say of the dead, "Oh, she would have wanted it that way," because they are usually talking so much sentimental nonsense. But I knew how Nanny Rose felt about me and about that coat, and about the two of us getting together sometime. "You'll wear it," she predicted. My grandmother's coat. My coat. It didn't—only weeks before, it couldn't—literally bring her closer to me. It was, after all, only a coat. But it brought its own consolations. Always it would recall for me her goodness and her generosity. I loved to reply simply, "My grandmother," when asked where the sleekly styled coat had come from. Things were that simple for her. All she wanted was to give me the coat off her back. Even her best one. Nothing Too Good....

Aggie's Declaration of Independence

by

Evelyn G. Kenney

Aggie sat in the back of Martin's car clutching her worn leather bag as they pulled out of the driveway. Her eyes drank in all the familiar surroundings because she knew she would not be coming back. It was important to commit to memory every picket of the fence, every shingle of the roof, even the rusty-colored mums that grew beside the path. There were twenty-seven pieces of slate leading to the front door and she knew the color and shape of every one. Her mind was keen. It wasn't any harder to remember the end of World War II, than to remember what she had for dinner the night before. Aggie knew she could file things away in her memory and retrieve them any time she wanted.

Her needs were of a physical nature: someone to do her wash, prepare her meals and tidy up a bit. If her legs were weak and her step was shaky it didn't matter too much, for it was the mind that was important. She had fallen a few times and, fortunately, was always able to pick herself up. But it was a signal to her that the time would come when she wouldn't be able to and that was when she decided to sell the house and make the move to the nursing home.

How she hated those words, nursing and home. After all, it wasn't nursing that she needed, it was just the idea of having someone nearby, of not being alone. She wasn't sick, just old. And home? She was leaving her home. The nursing home would never really be home to her, just a place to spend her later years.

The ride was long, but Aggie didn't mind. She was quite comfortable and the leaves were just beginning to turn. It was still her favorite time of year. Autumn, with its golden hues—a veritable palette of color. It always seemed to come as a renewal of determination, a time when she would come alive again.

Pam, her daughter-in-law, tried to make idle conversation and Aggie wished she would stop trying so hard.

A long time ago Aggie promised herself that no matter what the future held for her, she would never burden any of her children. That was how she was. She loved them all and she never doubted they loved her, too, but she never wanted to live with any of them.

Aggie knew she would decide for herself when it was time to leave her home. Perhaps the fact that Joe had been at the nursing home for several months helped to make her decision easier. Yet, after sixty years, she wondered why she hadn't really missed him too much when he had to go into the home. It wasn't that she didn't love him; she loved him then and she loved him now. Every week Aggie visited her husband and patiently listened to his complaints. He was a terrible patient and nothing had happened to change him. If anything, he was worse, more demanding and less tolerant than ever.

Aggie had delayed putting him into the home until her own health began to deteriorate and she simply could not, physically, give him the care he needed. He pleaded to stay with her and this made her feel all the more guilty. He told her she was selfish and he hurt her when he said that. It was an awful thing to say after all the care she had given him.

Still, it was a very hard decision to make, and she wondered if she would have been strong enough to make it alone. Her son, Martin, and his wife, Pam, stood by her decision and she was

23

thankful for that. Her other son, Timmy, and his family were out in California, but she knew she had their support as well.

Aggie also had a daughter, Jenny, but she wasn't sure just where she was. If she had one regret it was that she had stood by her husband when he disowned Jenny. He did it, he said, with good reason. For one thing, Jenny had married a Catholic and, to make matters worse, their son didn't like baseball. And if those weren't good enough reasons, he said, the mere fact that he had sired a girl would have been all the reason he needed to disown her since everyone knew that Joe was a man's man, and men should only sire sons.

Aggie's thoughts travelled back to the last time she had heard her daughter's voice. Fifteen years ago and Aggie still remembered the sound of it. For a moment she closed her eyes and rested her head back, trying to imagine how Jenny might look today. She even wondered if she would recognize her. Then a thin little smile crossed her lips and she whispered to herself, "Oh, yes I would. I would know my Jenny anywhere."

But that part of her life was over and it was a beautiful day. Aggie wasn't going to dwell on unpleasant thoughts. For however long it would be, today would begin a new part of her life. Most people her age shied away from talk of death or finality, but she never had, not when she was younger, and certainly not now. She looked upon life as a series of phases and death was the last phase.

It was Thursday, a strange day to begin anything. Usually things commenced on Mondays, sometimes even on Saturdays, but never on Thursdays. However, the closing on the house had been the day before and there was no point waiting. Everything was gone and she was a stranger in a house that now belonged to someone else. She really didn't want to stay a moment longer than she had to.

"We'll see you on Sunday, Mother," said Pam.

"How about dinner and a drive if the weather's nice?" joined in Martin.

But Aggie had her own ideas. She was all too familiar with the pattern. It reminded her of when someone dies and the first few weeks everyone calls and visits. Then, when you really need someone, they are gone. If she could help it, that wasn't going to happen to her. Take it slow.

"No, I think I would like to meet my new friends at the home," she answered, "and Sunday dinner is probably about the best way to do it. I don't think I want to make any plans right now. But please call me and we'll make plans in a few weeks."

"If that's the way you want it," said Pam.

And Martin added, "Maybe the Apple Festival at Mill Neck in October. We haven't missed a year since I was in high school."

"That's right. I forgot about that," said Aggie, as she made a mental note to circle the date on her calendar.

Soon they turned into the familiar horseshoe drive. The nursing home was essentially a large Victorian house which had been added onto, room by room, over the years. There was a front porch with a few rockers, all occupied by people who looked up from their knitting or reading as the car stopped in front of the steps. It was different coming here as a visitor. Now she was a guest and she would notice things she hadn't paid attention to before.

Martin opened the door and helped her out of the car. She walked up the stairs with Pam, and Martin followed them with her luggage. The other guests were curious. A few she recognized from all the times she had visited Joe.

"Nice to see you again," called out the lady with the knitting.

"Thank you, it's nice to see you, too," Aggie replied. It was good to see a friendly face. But she reminded herself to be cautious, not to respond too eagerly in the beginning. She had an uncanny way of sensing things in people, and it wasn't always a gift. Sometimes she knew she was too critical. Aggie had a different way of thinking about things than other people did. For instance, she always said, "Go by first impressions," while everyone else cautioned, "Don't go by first impressions."

As they entered the foyer, a young man ran past them to help Martin with her bags; his name was Tony. She remembered him bringing books for Joe and Joe telling him to take them away because he wasn't much of a reader. Joe liked to work with his hands in his shop, and if he couldn't do that he didn't care to do

25

anything else. The therapist brought puzzles and crafts for him, but he told her to give them to someone who would appreciate them more. It seemed like everything they attempted, he resisted, so finally they stopped trying and he just lay in his bed all day, staring at the ceiling. The wheelchair remained in the corner of his room and he never used it.

As Aggie watched Tony dash off, Miss Bonham came out of her office to greet Aggie.

"Welcome, Agnes," she said with her usual unaffected warmth. Aggie had always felt that Felicia Bonham was sincere and genuinely gracious. She wasn't a young woman, but compared to most of her guests, she appeared that way. Never very good at judging ages, Aggie supposed she was probably in her mid to late forties.

"Good to finally be here," replied Aggie with a smile.

"After all you have been through the past few weeks, I know you will enjoy the rest," said Miss Bonham. "Moving has to be one of the worst things a body can ever be made to endure." She turned to Martin and Pam. "Nice to see you again. As soon as they finish moving your father into the room, we'll go upstairs."

Aggie puzzled for a moment, as if she wasn't sure she should say anything. But if she didn't say anything now, it would be too late later on.

"Uh...Miss Bonham," she faltered.

Miss Bonham looked at Aggie, "Is something wrong?"

"Well, I just wondered why they would be moving Joe out of the room he was in?" Aggie's voice was barely audible.

Miss Bonham appeared to be taken aback. "We were moving him into *your* room, Agnes. That's what we usually do when we have married couples. Is there something wrong with that arrangement?"

For one brief moment Aggie almost said no. Sometimes it was easier to agree than to assert yourself. But easier wasn't always better and she was tired, tired of always doing what someone else wanted.

So Aggie stood as tall as she could and looked Miss Bonham directly in the eye. Her voice had taken on strength. "Yes, I'm

26

afraid there is something wrong with that arrangement, Miss Bonham. I do *not* want to share my room with my husband."

Martin and Pam looked shocked and Miss Bonham tried to reason with Aggie.

"We've already moved his belongings into your room. Everything has been moved but his bed, and they're moving that now, with him in it." Her calm, sweet voice had suddenly taken on a very acid tone.

Aggie waited for her to say, "Now, you wouldn't want us to move him out again after going to all that trouble, would you?" But she didn't, even though the inference was there.

How easy it would have been for Aggie to say forget about it. She was always a very considerate person, never one to cause extra work or bother for others. But this time, for the first, and possibly the last time in her life, she was declaring her own independence.

"Well, move them out," was Aggie's reply. "It's my room and you shouldn't have assumed I wanted to share it."

"Are you sure that's what you want, Ma?" Martin said as he struggled to understand. He was embarrassed for Miss Bonham, but he knew his mother was right. They should have asked her first.

Tears filled Aggie's eyes, but she was never more determined than she was at this moment. She took in a deep breath and said, "For more than sixty years I have shared a room and everything else in my life with Joe. I never minded because I loved him, and I still do. But I need someone to care for me now. I'm not strong enough to care for both of us. That's why we're here, Martin. Can you understand that?"

Pam spoke up after a long silence. "I think I understand that, Mom, and I think Martin does, too. But even if we didn't, it wouldn't matter. It has to be your decision."

A few hours later, after an exhausting day, Aggie had moved into her new room and it felt good just to kick off her shoes and relax. Aggie had spoken to Joe before Martin and Pam left and he pleaded with her to change her mind, but Aggie remained strong. If he wanted to visit he could. He could use the wheelchair; it had been his choice not to. Besides, she had to pass his room whenever she went downstairs to the dining room. So she would have to pass his room a few times a day anyway. They would visit, just as they had before Aggie moved to the home. But she wasn't going to be his caretaker ever again.

One day when Martin visited, he asked her—the way he usually did—if there was anything she needed. Usually she said no, or maybe she'd want some yarn if she was running low. But this time she asked him to buy her a red dress.

"A red dress?" He looked surprised. She had never asked for anything like that before. "Why do you want a red dress, Ma?"

"Well," she said, "I think about how things were between your father and me, and I never forgot the time I brought home a red dress. I think we were going to a New Year's Eve party. Anyway, when I put on the dress he got very angry, actually threw a fit. 'Take that dress off,' he yelled. So I asked, 'Why? Don't you like it?' And he said I looked like a streetwalker. I cried as though my heart would break.

"We never went to the party and I took the dress back to the store the next day or so. But, you know, Martin, all through the years I thought about that dress and I really would like to have a red dress before I die."

"Oh, Ma," Martin said, "you're not gettin' ready to die. But if you really want a red dress, I'll ask Pam to pick out one for you."

Sure enough, a few days later, Pam brought not one, but two dresses. "Why two?" Aggie asked in surprise.

"Well," Pam explained, "one is about as red as you can get— a real dynamite red—and it's silky and dressy. The other is not quite so red, more like a burgundy, and it's polyester, so you can wash it out and hang it up to dry. In case you wanted something more practical."

But even as she said it, Pam knew Aggie had had enough of being practical. "I'll take the red," Aggie said as she reached out for it.

"Don't you want to try it first?" Pam asked.

"Nope. It'll be just fine," Aggie said. "In fact, I'll wear it down to dinner tonight."

On the way downstairs, she stopped to see Joe. He almost

28

dropped his fork when she stuck her head in the door, followed by her red-dressed body.

"Where do you think you're goin'?" he asked suspiciously.

"To dinner," she said. "Care to join me?"

"Nope," he answered, shaking his head the way he always did. "If you want to make a fool of yourself, you don't need me with you to do it."

"Fine. Enjoy your dinner," she replied, undaunted.

When Aggie entered the dining room every eye was upon her as she found her way to her table. Tony, the young man who helped out at the home, poured her water. "You sure look pretty," he said. "And in that dress you remind me of a lady I know, named Jenny."

And so Agnes had her own room and she could wear red anytime she wanted. But the best was yet to come. She was going to see Jenny again, and if Joe wanted to share her joy she would give him the chance, but she wasn't expecting any miracles. Just finding Jenny's address seemed miracle enough.

Aggie's Declaration of Independence was now complete.

The Kiss

by

Frank Finale

My wife and I, in the throes of the January blahs, had just finished eating supper. We were clearing the table and trying to
avoid stepping into each other's path in our tiny kitchen apartment when she walked over to the steamed-up window. Using a
dish rag, she wiped off some of the condensation and peered out.
"Look at it snowing!" she called to me.

Rushing to the window to join her, I looked out and saw a
steady stream of flakes in the street light. Opening the window,
some snow whirled in from the darkness. The fresh, cold smell
left me giddy. I had looked before and didn't see a thing. Now
the dark cracks of the walkways were filled with white. Ghosts of
snow descended on the bones of the three maple trees outside
our window and shrubs were little white hillocks.

The town's sanitation department had been caught off
guard. One lone car, like some bewildered beetle, was feeling its
way up the avenue.

We turned toward each other and caught each other's
thought. It had been years since we had gone for a walk in the
snow just for the sheer joy of it. "Let's do it!" we both seemed to
cry at once.

We layered ourselves with clothes—long johns, flannels,

sweaters—and topped everything off with hooded coats. Looking and feeling like Arctic explorers minus the dog sled, we abandoned the dirty dishes and set out from the steam-heated, oven-warmed kitchen into the night.

A vast whiteness dwarfed us. Avenues had lost their names. We walked past the Chatfields' yard, where a hapless Chevy pickup sat on the blocks of its final resting place. The snow had pulled a sheet over its rusted body. We walked past the DeGiorgios', whose once brilliant rose garden was now abloom in white. We trudged down to the muffled roar of the ocean three blocks away.

Running across Ocean Avenue, we plunged into a thigh-high snowdrift and tumbled out, laughing so hard our tears mixed with the snow melting on our red faces. We crunched our way up to the boardwalk, the cold air burning our lungs as we gasped for breath.

Standing near the shore's edge, in the night, there were few points of reference. The only sounds were the soft shushing of the snow and the harsh hissing of the sea. There were no boundaries. Looking up into the swirling night, I grew dizzy and felt as though I would fall off the end of the earth if I did not grab onto something solid. Gripping the iron railing of the boardwalk, I looked at my wife. Between the flakes I could see her red hood. Although we were a couple of feet from each other, she could barely hear me call out, "Let's go back."

She agreed. What began as a walk in the snow was rapidly becoming a survival mission. As we were going, she pulled me into an alcove by a boarded-down hotdog stand. There—unexpectedly—she kissed me.

The white balloons of our breath held no words, but I still remember that simple kiss. Time seemed to stop. Her breath tasted of wintergreen and her lips were moist against mine. The gloom of the alcove lit up. The jasmine scent of her perfume filled my senses and washed away the dank odor of that shelter. Our boots squeaked as we swayed back and forth. Though our faces were numb and the cold and the dark engulfed us, this one sweet kiss seemed to prove our existence. Outside the alcove, the snow

31

seethed. Abandoning ourselves to our own weather, we kissed again. I felt at peace with myself and everything around me.

But then it was time to leave. The snow was deeper now and fell more heavily and quickly. No cars were out, so we had the joyful experience of galumphing down the middle of the avenue without having to worry about traffic. The shells of our ears held an ocean sound, our fingers, feet, and faces tingling like a thousand stars. Wind wolves howled around us and followed us to our door, where we left them. We stayed up into the early morning hours, watched old movies on TV, and made love as the radiator hissed and knocked far into the night.

I had never felt so alive.

Hooked on Mahogany

by

Mike Lipstock

He was an old man who brought his poles and tackle to the dock each day and loved to fish. He would sit in the warm Florida sun after a lifetime of winter snows and watch the movement in the water that swarmed around him. His tired old eyes would watch the ripples in the water, which sounded like the strings of a harp. At dusk he would hold fast to his line and watch the flocks of white ibis rushing back before the sun set. To where? Perhaps beyond the sea to a paradise only birds knew

The egrets and cormorants, in a fluttering of color, usually announced the end of the day. Were they off to a bird paradise also? How hard they worked, diving beneath the sea for a meal and stalking on tiptoe lest the insects hear them.

He fished and he watched.

Through trial and error he had learned the feeding habits of each fish. His favorite was the sheepshead with teeth so strong they could crush barnacles. For them the old man needed special bait. He would go to the creeks at low tide and dig up the small fiddler crabs that lived in the sand at the edge of the shore, filling his bucket to the brim every day. The sheepshead couldn't resist

33

them. Other bait helped him harvest all types of fish from this beautiful portion of sea.

And then a flock of birds became his constant companions—the pelicans. He couldn't help but love them. He was fascinated with their flight. Never could there be such a grand sight as a squad of pelicans coming in from high altitude and sweeping down to the very edge of the sea, just inches from the water. Heads held high, wings fixed, and their bodies streamlined for maximum glide. Suddenly they would go into a steep climb...and then the great miracle! With wings thrust out and bills plunging ahead like armed weapons, they went into vertical dives at break-neck speed, cutting through the water like missiles and emerging with throats gorged with wriggling fish. At that tremendous speed he marveled that they didn't crush their wings.

The fledglings were all dressed in their new brown feathers, gangly, and still in flight training. But the adults...ah, the adults. He couldn't take his eyes off them. In the air they used a pelican code and rode the thermal currents in perfect V formation. They always took him back to his war days and reminded him of the bombers returning from a combat mission.

And still he fished and watched.

There were four or five pelicans that would sit with great patience next to him on the dock and wait for the next fish he would toss their way. They had curious eyes with yellow irises and black pu-pils. Their bodies were brown and the huge shovels for mouths were all identical. All of their large arched necks were white, but one alone was different. He seemed older, wiser, something like himself. He was the one with the deep brown neck. He sat to closer to him than the rest.

And still the old man fished and watched.

Some days the old man would come even if the tide was out, for he had patience and a lot of time. Soon his brown-necked friend would sidle up to him and they both would wait for the day's first catch. In his mind, he named the pelican "Mahogany" and couldn't wait for him to swoop in and gently land at his side.

He was using squid for bait that morning and quickly hooked a fish that brought him to his feet. His light pole was bending almost in half. It had to be a Jack Crevalle, the bulldog of the sea. He jammed the pole under his still powerful arm and played him. Sure enough, out of the corner of his eye he could see Mahogany glide without a flutter of wings across the calm sea and suddenly drop daintily at his side to watch the struggle going on.

The old man had the line out and was working him in. He looked at his friend and gently spoke to him as an equal, "Where have you been, my friend? You sit and wait while my tired arms twist and pull for your breakfast! Did you go with the white ibis last night to your secret nesting grounds? You look at me with your yellow eyes and I'm never sure if you approve. But sit and wait, Mahogany. If this fish doesn't break my arm, you'll have a fine meal."

The fish was sapping the old man's strength, but it finally broke the water and he could see that it was a hefty jack. As soon as he landed it he was surrounded by a wave of young white-necked pelicans. They were in a frenzy for the jack, but calm old Mahogany just sat there and waited.

The old man drove the others away and bucketed the struggling jack. Mahogany never budged when the rest flew off. The old man cut the fish into chunks that the pelican could catch. He tossed the pieces into Mahogany's cavernous mouth and, when he finished the last piece, the bird gave the old man a nod of satisfaction and a nudge with his huge beak. They were a couple of old timers hanging on.

And still he fished and watched.

At twilight the old man looked up and saw a flurry of egrets that looked like thousands of white butterflies fluttering away somewhere beyond land's end. Across the cove he saw the pelicans returning from yet another expedition. Like old bombers with outstretched wings, they circled a cluster of casserina pines that grew almost out of the water. One by one the great birds lowered their flap feathers in midair, stalled, and with webbed landing gear down, shuddered to a halt on the flimsy trembling branches.

At the very top of the tallest tree he could see the brown neck of Mahogany preening his wings. Suddenly the bird fixed his gaze on the old man, who doffed his hat in tribute and half whispered, "See you in the morning, my friend."

When he came to the dock in the morning, the aged bird was waiting and the old man spoke to him seriously. "Do you eat catfish? Okay, we'll go to the cove today and see if you like what I catch."

He moved his gear and put some cut mullet on the hooks. In a minute he had a bite and held on for dear life. Something was tearing his arm out of the socket. Mahogany flew over to the new spot, his eyes and erect feathers signaled his excitement. The old man landed a monster of a catfish. He was very cautious with the dorsal and pectoral fins; each was barbed, a hidden stiletto capable of tearing the skin to the bone. The old man dispatched the brute and nudged a piece toward his friend, but the millennia had programmed the bird to be wary of those barbs. He snubbed his beak at the fish and walked away from his breakfast.

The old man loved catfish and knew just how to dress them for a tasty meal. He was also curious if Mahogany would take them defanged. With a sharp fillet knife he removed the spikes and filleted the fish while the bird watched his every move. He tossed him a few chunks and the usually ravenous pelican turned and again walked away, following his innate instincts.

As the sun crept up to the midday position, the two of them dozed in the warmth of the winter sun. It was late in the afternoon when the old man again attracted a bevy of young pelicans searching for a meal. They all sat near Mahogany and waited for the old man to throw them a fish.

His pole bent and the birds knew immediately what was going to happen. A few stayed on the dock, but the others were already in the water ready to pluck the fish from his line. Trouble was brewing and more wings fluttered above him as his fight went on. Suddenly the fish broke water and there was a mad dash of birds battling for the fish that was still hooked to the line. The old man was afraid to pull it up. If they took it they would get the hook as well. He kept the fish under water and waited for the right moment. When it came, he pulled hard and watched the birds slash each other with their sword-like bills. As he reeled in the fish, it dropped from the line. To his horror he saw the loose hook rip into the bystander, Mahogany.

The man's emotions were so affected that he could feel the hook in his own flesh. He winced! God, what had he done? His friend had the hook imbedded deep in his back and for a moment he could feel the pelican's weight hanging from the pole. He cut the line and the bird immediately flew off with fifteen feet of line dangling from his wounded body. The old man's mind raced. Could Mahogany survive with the deeply imbedded hook? Would it rust? Would it infect him?

The next morning, the old man left his poles at home and walked back to the dock looking for Mahogany, but he was gone. No one had seen him. The poles remained in the house because the old man no longer fished. He just searched for the bird with the dark brown neck.

And then one day he looked up into the steel gray sky and watched a small group of pelicans come in over the water, stretch their mighty wings and dive bomb the tiny cove that was alive with small fish. Again and again they went into their steep dives and scooped up wriggling fish that dripped from their huge mouths. Mahogany was leading the pack, still trailing fifteen feet of nylon line. Now, for the first time since he'd hooked the pelican, the old man got his pole and once again fished and watched.

He fished near a forest of mangrove whose twisted roots sheltered a variety of fish. He tossed his line near the edge and soon had a flaming red snapper tugging on the light pole. Sure enough the big bird with the long leash showed his confidence and dropped down not more than a foot away. The old man could see the golden hook in the very center of his back. He held the fish and coaxed him even closer. The huge head was close to his lap when he tossed the fish. Mahogany lunged and the old man clasped him to his chest as he struggled. He ran with Mahogany to a friend's boat and, with a pair of thin pliers, they pulled the hook out in minutes.

Mahogany flew up as soon as the old man let him loose. Those huge wings pumped a few times and then he went into a glide. The old bird banked in a wide turn and dropped gently to the dock, this time almost in the man's lap. The old man looked into his yellow eyes and smiled. It was nice to have him back again.

He looked out to sea—not a ripple, not a sound. The sun was up and everything glowed. In minutes the still blue water turned to gold.

Yes, he thought, it would be a good winter. They would fish side by side and watch the cormorants, ibis and blue heron fly over to their own very special spot. Maybe he would even stroke the brown old neck and the two of them would watch the teeming ocean life from their own very special dock. He smiled and looked at his friend, who stared back at him with his wise old yellow eyes.

Black Stockings

by

Elsie A. Schmied

I loved being a student nurse in Milwaukee, Wisconsin. I met new people and I learned how the human body functions and what to do when things go wrong. And I felt ten feet tall when a patient said, "Thank you for the back rub. You made me feel so much better."

I was living a dream I'd had since kindergarten.

The life of a student nurse in the mid-1940s was far from glamorous. The food we ate was mostly starch and there was never enough to satisfy the appetite of a growing girl. I used to hide a jar of peanut butter in my dresser and eat it by the spoon-ful just to fill up.

Our routine was to work eight hours, go to class for three or four more, and then study. I was always tired as a result, ofttimes falling asleep over my books and waking up with a crick in my neck. On my two half-days off duty, I studied or slept and lived in constant fear I'd never learn enough to be a good nurse.

In our sixth week, we went on the hospital floors. That was when we started wearing our uniforms. These were sand-colored, belted, with white collar and short sleeves. The two patch pockets were always lumpy, bulging with pens, scissors, and note pads.

And the outfit was decidedly unfashionable in other ways as

39

well, sagging halfway between the knees and ankles at a time when other eighteen-year-olds wore knee-length skirts.

Accessories? Well, we had to wear cotton undergarments to prevent sparking an explosion of anesthetic gases in the operating room! I tolerated the cotton slips, but I detested the hideous black stockings that we had to wear. These, I thought, were the final indignity.

And so hard to find! A week before I had to wear them, my folks and I searched the stores. It turned out that black stockings were as rare as chocolate bars during the war. In desperation, my mother dyed six pairs of tan cotton hose black.

I was ready.

My first patient contact was to be evening care for three patients. This meant helping with their toileting needs, washing hands and faces, and brushing their teeth. We, who had never touched a stranger, had to wash their backs and even give back rubs with rubbing alcohol and talcum powder. Even worse, everyone knew we were only probationers with hair nets, not nurses caps, on our heads.

I was so nervous my hands were wet. The armpits of my uniform were soaked within ten minutes.

My first three hours were like three years.

Somehow all my patients ate their suppers and I finished their care. The head nurse inspected the ward and found dust on the base of one over-bed table. Nonetheless, she said I was adequate and dismissed me for the evening. Relieved, I hurried to the nurses' home.

Safe in my room I kicked my black shoes off. The linings were damp with perspiration. I peeled my garter belt and stockings off; my feet were black as coal. I hung my uniform in the closet and tried to scrub and scrub the color off my feet. Five minutes before study hall I dried my gray feet, pulled on white ankle socks and saddle shoes, and dashed downstairs.

For two whole months my feet ranged in color from dead black to ash gray. The black stayed on the body of the hose, but the

40

color on the feet of the stockings transferred to my own feet and the lining of my shoes, until everything was a dirty gunmetal color.

Slowly my feet faded. Best of all, my wonderful father scoured the city during his lunch hours until he found some black rayon stockings in a hosiery store downtown. He gave me three pairs as a Christmas gift. How I treasured them.

During our second year we met students from other hospitals, most of whom also were plagued with black stockings. One exception were the lucky students from a fancy east-side hospital; they wore *white* shoes and stockings. Our class talked it over and agreed: white stockings and shoes would be *far* more attractive with our uniforms. We petitioned the Director of Nursing. She refused to listen. "Tradition," she said.

Later that year we spent three months at Children's Hospital. For a week each student was assigned to the Milk Lab, making formula and sterilizing bottles. On my second day I carried an open pan of freshly sterilized nipples, awash in a sea of boiling water, across the room to the counter where we capped the formula bottles. Still wearing my dyed stockings, I slipped and slid like a burlesque comic, the water splashing and scalding both my feet. I received a reprimand, then hobbled for a week. But worst of all, I had those horrible gray feet again for days, until the skin finally peeled off.

Counting down to the end of our 1,095 student days, I dreamed of white stockings and fashionably short uniforms. But, unbeknownst to me, I hadn't seen the end of black stockings.

One evening while on duty, a visitor handed me a package, thanking me for the care of his wife through her pneumonia crisis. We weren't supposed to accept gifts from patients, but he gave one to every student on the unit and the head nurse said we could keep them.

Inside the box were three pairs of the first nylon stockings I had ever seen: sheer as cobwebs and seamed up the back. Our grateful visitor owned a hosiery store. I wore these precious black nylons on Sundays until graduation.

Meanwhile, our class bought our fitted, short-skirted uniforms and much-desired white shoes and stockings long before the big day. On August 28, 1947, our class of 21 young women paraded proudly into the church in our crisp, shapely white uniforms, white stockings and shoes, and starched white caps to receive our school pins on graduation day. Black stockings would henceforth be a thing of the past.

The following month a young Frenchman named Christian Dior showed his first collection, "The New Look." He featured longer skirts about halfway between the knee and ankle. His models pranced down the runway wearing black stockings with their pumps. And I thought, *Sometimes you just can't win.*

But I never could bring myself to wear "The New Look."

A Sprig of Thyme

by

Dorothy Winslow Wright

We were northerners, new to the southern town in the heart of
the Shenandoah Valley—a Virginia town surrounded by mountains with air as sweet as honeysuckle in the spring. As welcoming
as the environs were, it didn't take me long to realize that New
Englanders were "damn Yankees" and that the Civil War was not
a closed issue.

Bud, my husband, learned to say "ah reckon" when dealing
with his co-workers, while I found "y'all" slipping into my vocabulary as easily as grits slipped into my cooking. The gap was closing, but not enough to make me feel a totally welcome neighbor.

When Molly and Clay moved onto our street, I expected the
same distancing. Clay—Richmond born and bred—was as southern as Robert E. Lee. But not Molly—she was a statuesque Iowan
with a rollicking, whopping laugh.

In the early spring, when Molly and I first became friends,
we often sat in the backyard while our babies toddled around the
budding apple trees. I said, "Wouldn't it be nice to have a rock
garden with violets and columbine, and maybe lady slippers."

"There's no way you'll grow lady slippers in this soil," Molly
allowed, "but you can find things that will grow here down by the
river. All the violets you want or bleeding hearts...."

"Hold on, Molly. I have a baby. Remember?" I interrupted. "This yard is headed for swings and a sandbox."

"A rock garden doesn't take up that much room and children like gardens," she replied. "But how would you know, being a city slicker."

Molly was right. The only gardening I had done was on a third floor windowsill of a Boston apartment building.

That evening Bud loosened the soil under the apple tree while I ambled along the alley picking up rocks. The next day he presented me with a flat of velvety pansies—yellow, dark-eyed pansies as bright as the sun itself. I planted them after supper.

Molly inspected my efforts. "It's a good start," she said, "but you need more rocks—bigger ones—and some herbs."

"Herbs?" I said. "You mean like parsley?"

"Among others," she nodded. "You know how to cook with herbs, don't you? Or are you Bostonians no-nonsense purists?" Although she smiled, I sensed something in her voice that told me she wasn't sure how much teasing I could take about my beloved Massachusetts home.

"Well, I do put sage in my turkey stuffing and chop parsley to garnish my boiled potatoes." I leaned over and picked up a pansy. "I love these. They're friendly —friendlier than the neighbors."

Molly raised her eyebrows. "What about me?"

"You're different," I said.

I hadn't meant to bring up the subject; it sounded whiny, but once I started, I couldn't stop. Everything came flooding out—my loneliness, homesickness, how different things were in the South. How, in short, I felt every bit the condemned "damn Yankee."

"So what's new?" Molly said. There was no denial, yet with those three words I knew she understood my feelings. Maybe they echoed hers.

The next Saturday, tall rangy Clay meandered up through the backyard carrying a dirt-smudged newspaper. He was dressed in denim overalls, not looking the least like the scientific research maven that drove to work each day.

"Molly said you're starting a rock garden," he said, "so I reckoned you could use these. They look a mite spindly, but they're healthy." He crushed a leaf in his fingers. It smelled tangy. "Lemon verbena, and these are chives and thyme. If you add a sprig of thyme when you're cooking carrots, it'll take the woodiness out."

He squatted down and showed me where and how to plant the herbs, then stood and wiped his muddy hands on his overalls. "If you wear jeans," he said eyeing my crisp tan pedal pushers, "you can get as dirty as I do. You can dig right in and not worry about the dirt. It's good for the garden—having y'all loose like that."

He didn't say it would be good for me, too, but I knew that's what he meant. I needed to shed some of my white-gloved Boston attitude to fit in with the local folks.

I sat on the grass and began to dig with my new silvery trowel. I ignored the dirt on my hands as I tamped the ground around each herb. Those plants were going to make it!

Bud came out. "You've got enough dirt on your face to start another garden," he said, grinning.

I was surprised. "I do?" I asked. Then I recovered. "Sorry about that. But look, Bud. Clay gave me all these herbs. Chives, thyme, and lemon verbena." I snapped off a leaf and let him sniff it.

"Hmm," he said. "Looks like your new boyfriend did all right by you."

I made the expected face, but I didn't mind being teased. It was good to have friends again—and I knew that Molly and Clay would be special ones.

The town became a friendlier place as my little rock garden began to flourish. Candytuft, mint, creeping phlox tumbled down the bank, blossoming as our family blossomed in the welcoming climate.

Clay showed me how to prune the herbs when they became leggy; how to divide chives when a clump was too thick. When he acquired a new herb, he shared it with me. When I came by some columbine, I split it with him.

When the thyme wandered over the rocks, I snipped it and

45

gave it to the neighbors for their carrots. I gave them chives for party sandwiches, oregano for spaghetti sauce, rosemary for their roast pork. They gave me cucumbers, eggplants, and invited me in for coffee.

A few years later, when a company transfer sent our family two hundred miles away, I planted a sprig of thyme in a small pot so it would survive in the motel until we moved into our house. Once settled in, Clay's thyme graced our driveway.

A rooted sprig of that same thyme was the first plant set into the slope behind a newer home in a northern city—a slope not too different from the one beneath the old apple tree in Virginia. My thyme became a city dweller as I was again by then, but a city dweller who liked to dig in the earth on a dew-wet bank breathing in the pungent scent of thyme.

When Molly died, I knelt by my garden at the hour of her funeral. As I pulled weeds from around the thyme's rootstock, I was aware that there would have been no rootstock at all if Molly hadn't heard my cry of loneliness so many years ago. And if Clay, a proper southern gentleman, hadn't ambled my way with an armful of scrawny herbs.

Clay and I are an ocean and a continent apart these days, but we write to one another now and then. Sometimes he sends me lavender.

One Last Snake Story

by

Kristina D. Baguley

I see a snake. Rather, I see the tips of the grass shudder in a serpentine path. There is a snakeness in that motion. It reminds me of my grandfather, not because he had anything in common with snakes, but because of the way he would dispatch one.

He'd hear our cries of "Snake!" and he'd come out of the house slowly, cradling his rifle and fumbling for his glasses. The old man would walk right up to that snake, close enough to make us wonder if he didn't see it. Without a word, he'd chamber a round and slowly raise that rifle butt to his shoulder. He'd squint down the rifle barrel, the muzzle almost within the snake's striking range. And the gun's muzzle would wobble about, betraying my grandfather's struggle with age and trifocals. Or so I thought.

After what seemed like many whole minutes to a small child holding her breath, the gun would bark and the snake would writhe only once more. My grandfather would lower the gun as slowly as he had raised it and turn back to whatever project he had left, leaving us kids to discover that the snake's head was shot clean off. I never saw Grandad shoot at anything but snakes, but I never saw him miss a snake either. Looking at those dead snakes, it was easy to believe the story that people told about him, that as a young man he would shoot holes in coins thrown into the air.

My father taught me to shoot a rifle when I was ten, and I got good enough for my brothers to stop saying "not bad, for a girl" and start betting on me against their friends. Still, I was not good enough to hit flying coins or shoot heads off snakes. Grandad wasn't telling me how, either. I'd ask, and he'd smile and stare off into space for a while, and then start telling me one snake story or another from his younger years. He had a lot of those, having grown up along the Mississippi River. And he spoke very slowly, more slowly than others who hail from Louisiana. My mother said it was because he'd been nearly killed with gas during the Great War. Consequently, just one of his snake stories, with its winding turns, would use up all my ability to sit still. So, question still unanswered, I would go back out with the rifle and practice more on paper targets and cans and wonder if it was just a matter of learning how to hit moving things.

My father's gun book told of "leading" a moving target, so I practiced sighting on and leading moving objects with the gun unloaded. I never knew whether I was "leading" completely wrong or only a little bit right or what, since the only moving thing I hated enough to chamber a round on was a snake. And they would laugh at me and slither away when I missed them. After a while I gave up on ever hitting a snake at all, let alone hitting one in the head.

But one day in my sixteenth summer, I found myself face to face with a snake and my grandfather's rifle in my hands. I pictured Grandad walking up to a snake with that gun and once more I wondered what in that picture I had missed, the secret difference between shooting snakes and just shooting at snakes. I saw his slow, deliberate aim again. And then I saw a twelve-year-old girl rehearsing shouldering a rifle and squeezing off quick shots over and over.

Very slowly I shouldered the rifle and began looking for the snake's head in the sights. The steadier I tried to hold the rifle, the more the muzzle wobbled. Surely the snake would strike while I wavered, or slither away. But I suppressed the twitch in my trigger finger and waited for a better picture, trying to track the snake's weaving head, trying to judge how much lead I needed.

48

And then, abruptly, the picture was perfect: the snake fixated on the wobbling muzzle and began to follow it with his head. I didn't have to aim at all, just wait until he joined the dance. It was so easy, I almost lowered the gun and walked away. But I had to know for sure. I pulled the trigger; the snake jerked once. His head was blown away.

I took that snake up by the house and hung it on the garden fence near where my grandfather worked every evening.

That night, Grandad and I sat together in the kitchen after everyone else had left the table. I knew he'd been out to the garden, but his eyesight had gotten so bad that I wondered if he had missed the dead snake. I wanted to tell him what I'd done, to show him that I'd finally learned his secret, but I was sixteen and bragging was something only little kids did. So I waited, like I had waited to pull the trigger that afternoon.

Finally he spoke. "Someone kilt a snake and hung 'im up." I waited for the inevitable snake story, but instead he told the story of shooting the coin thrown up in the air. A fellow had challenged him to try it. He was lucky and somehow—he never knew how—he hit it the very first try. He kept that damaged coin in his pocket—a lucky piece—for a long time. People would hear the story and, not believing, bet him that he couldn't really do it. He'd pull out that coin and people would withdraw their bet. He never had to shoot at another flying coin.

I asked him if he still had that coin. "Lost it in the War," was all he said. He never told war stories, so I didn't ask how. Instead, I watched him steady himself with the stair railing with each step he took as he made his way toward his bedroom. I imagined that he had lost the coin and its luck in the trenches in France, right before his unit got gassed.

He wouldn't have told me about the coin if he hadn't known I shot that snake. Years later, I watch the grass undulate in this snake's wake and treasure the seed of reality that grows into tall tales.

The Pulse of Saturday Night

by

Sonia Walker

Memories of the old dance hall
are sealed in the mind of
a middle-aged bopper
who remembers the magic
of Saturday night
many years ago when her
date appeared before
the door whistling the
latest tune while combing
his slick hair,
looking handsome in his
plaid jacket and freshly
polished white bucks.

The rag-top chevy had a Saturday
night shine, loud music playing
from its AM radio while both
sat close together,
his arm around her
pony-tailed shoulder,

they laughed in love as he
peeled rubber at the traffic light,
rushing to meet the gang at Wally's
Drive-in for burgers and shakes,
and then on their way to a night
of be-bop-a-loopa.

Boarded windows, faded paint,
a fallen sign, and unmowed grass
are yesterday's memories of a time
when "going steady" and "necking"
were favorite things to do;
she stops and stares at the
old dance hall recapturing
the pulse of Saturday night
which gives blueberry feelings to
her well-seasoned heart.

The Day the War Ended

by

Claudio G. Segrè

For as long as I could remember, people talked about the day when the war would end. By the spring of 1945, as I was finishing third grade, I sensed that the great day was approaching. Every day on the noon news, we followed the Allied race across Germany toward Berlin. In May the Germans surrendered. In the Pacific the Americans captured island after island and began bombing Japan regularly.

We lived in Los Alamos then, high in the mountains of New Mexico, where my father worked as a physicist. I noticed that he was gone for a few days in May, and again in July. He was doing his work, my mother said. He had been "in the desert," my father said when he returned. I wondered why physicists did their work in the desert. Did his job have something to do with the end of the war?

I wondered how wars ended. Did the enemies just stop fighting one day? Or was there one grand final battle, or one super bombing raid—the kind I sometimes drew in my war pictures—when our side, the American side, blew up all our enemies? How would people feel on the day the war ended?

It would be like recess at school, I decided. I would run around yelling and screaming, pushing and hitting, as my friends and I did when we first raced out into the schoolyard. I had a toy gun that fired paper rolls and made a noise like caps. I would certainly shoot that. I pictured a grand, all-American picnic.

Grown-ups—maybe even my mother and father—would relax. The most important leaders, like the President or the generals, would give fiery speeches. People would sing songs, wave American flags. At night the sky would fill with exploding, cascading fireworks. I would gorge myself with watermelon and hotdogs.

At the picnic, my mother (my father would be busy talking to his colleagues) would order me to calm down, to behave myself. But from her voice, from the way she turned back to talking with the other mothers, I knew that she didn't really mean it.

I imagined there would be a parade with heroes in uniform wearing their medals. They would look something like Barry Blake or Dave Dawson, the heroes in my war adventure books. They were all young, handsome, with shining white teeth. They wouldn't wear glasses, as I did.

And then the Great Day arrived. The week before came the news of the atomic bombs, first on Hiroshima on August 6, then on Nagasaki on August 9. At last, late in the afternoon on August 14, the official word came over the radio: "The Japanese have surrendered. The Second World War has come to an end." The radio announcer's voice sounded unusually deep, solemn, final, as if the President, or somehow even God, had given him the word directly.

This was the great day. I could see that people were gathering outside in the street. I wanted to wear shorts and tennis shoes. My mother made me put on blue jeans or patched corduroys and the brown high-topped shoes I hated. "We live in the mountains," she reminded me. Even in the middle of August, it could be cold.

Like our neighbors, the Allens, my parents and I gathered outside on our porch, just at the top of the stairs. I leaned over the balcony and looked down on our neighbors, the Olmsteads and the Perrys, on the families in the other complexes down the street. I had my cap gun. Everybody was screaming, "Yay, the war's over! The war's over!"

Like everyone else, I yelled, "The war's over!" I held my cap gun over my head, as if the noise would be too much for my ears. "The war's over!" I yelled. Bang! To augment the sound of my gun, I also yelled, "Bang!" I yelled again: "Yay, the war's over!" For good measure, I added, "And we won!"

My parents watched approvingly. I knew it was what they and their friends wanted to hear. I knew it was what the neighbors' kids were yelling, what the radio, like a broken record, announced over and over.

I knew I was yelling what I should be yelling, but secretly I had my doubts.

War had provided me and my friends with many grand adventures. In the woods in back of our house, we played fighter pilots, we were bombardiers on raids over Berlin, we drove tanks, we commanded battleships. We smeared our faces with a little dirt and like commandos snuck up on each other. But we knew that war was bad; peace was good. Our parents and teachers said so; the President said so; the heroes in my adventure books said so. Too many people, civilians and soldiers, men, women, and even children, who had nothing to do with the fighting, got hurt or even killed. In magazines I had seen pictures of bombed cities. In some cases nothing was left except the bare walls of buildings, and sometimes not even that—just piles of scattered, broken bricks.

Even my mother yelled a bit. "Hooray! The war is over!" My mother, in a plain skirt and cotton blouse, looked genuinely happy. My father just smiled. He was a small man and he was wearing his little dark-rimmed glasses so that he looked like the smartest kid in the class.

I wanted my parents to scream, to dance, to sing, to jump around. This was the great day, wasn't it? I set the example. I shrieked, wildly, hysterically. I jumped up and down. I fired my gun. The more I fired it, the sillier I felt. This great day called for resonant, thunderous "bangs," for ear-shattering "booms" that rolled and echoed off the mountain peaks. But now that I listened, I heard only "Pop! Pop!"

"The war's over! The war's over!" I screamed a couple of dozen times. My throat began to feel dry and scratchy; it hurt. My father looked bored; my mother had stopped yelling. There

54

didn't seem to be anything more to do or to say. I glanced at the stand of pine trees across the street, at the outline of the water tower up the hill. We were still here, still in the mountains, in the wilds of New Mexico. I wondered if I'd been screaming at nothing more than the trees, the wind and the mountains. Now my father looked annoyed; my mother looked ready to go inside. Where was the picnic, the grand celebration, the parade of heroes, the President?

Inside we went, my mother to washing some dishes, my father to reading the newspaper or doing calculations with his slide rule. The war was over and life went on, I discovered.

At least I was happy about one thing: the war had come to an all-American ending. "We," the Americans, the "good guys," invented the super weapon, the atomic bomb. With one grand and terrible blast, we had crushed our enemies.

But the more I thought about that all-American ending, the more questions I had. The super weapon, I knew, had been created in large part right here in Los Alamos, where I was living. Yet this was no all-American project. I thought of my father; I thought of all the people I knew who worked with him. They were nothing like the all-American heroes I had pictured at a victory parade. Many were Germans and Hungarians, Swiss and French, Italians and English. They all spoke with thick accents—even the ones from England. Instead of crisp uniforms they wore rumpled suits or jackets; some were balding and many wore glasses.

Bit by bit, I learned about what my father had been doing. The more I learned, the less all-American it sounded. In May, I learned long afterward, he had witnessed a practice test of the bomb with conventional explosives. Then, on July 15, he had been at Alamogordo for the first real bomb test.

It had been hot in the desert, he said. He had seen many scorpions and Gila monsters. The night before there had been a tremendous thunderstorm. Halfway through the night, he had been awakened by an unearthly noise. When he got up to investigate, he found dozens of frogs croaking love songs to each other in a mud hole. Would real all-American heroes pay attention to frogs in a mud hole? I wondered.

55

I felt better when I pictured him at the test site. There, like a commando, he lay flat on the sand. I imagined my father's suspense and anxiety.

For some days afterwards, I pondered the great day when the war ended. I was glad that the war was over, and that we had won. Still, I felt disappointed—even vaguely cheated. I wished I'd seen at least one ruined building or a dead soldier—preferably an enemy one. I had drawn so many pictures of aerial dogfights and of burning tanks that I wished I'd seen at least one real one. I saw pictures of the big victory parades in New York, and I was sorry I missed them.

I wondered what it would be like without the great drumbeat of the war in the background of our lives. What new games would I play? In place of war scenes, what new pictures would I draw?

Most of all, I wasn't sure anymore about all-American heroes, the kind I read about in my comic books or in my Barry Blake adventure stories, or the kind I'd imagined in the victory parade. Were there any like them in real life? Could it be that the real heroes who brought the war to an end were more like my father, with his delight over lovesick frogs?

Here, Chick, Chick, Chick

by

Jane Hill Purtle

One morning in March during the Great Depression, Ruby and
Russell were getting their garden ready for planting. They were
newlyweds and expecting their first baby. They borrowed Uncle
Tom Moore's wagon to haul manure from Ruby's papa's barn lot.
This was their first garden and they intended to make it a good
one. The red clay hill where they lived in East Texas was poor land,
but everybody knows what good manure will do for poor land.

They left the house about nine o'clock. Old Prince, the
horse they got from Mr. Roosevelt's "help-the-farmer program,"
pulled the wagon right along on the muddy road, and except for
Ruby's growling stomach, she felt good.

"Whoa, Prince," Russell called as they pulled up in the barnyard. "You okay, Ruby?"

"I'm fine. Just a little empty. My bowl of oatmeal's already disappeared," she answered.

"This is sure fine manure. It's good of your papa to let us
have it. It ought to grow some good potatoes and beans," Russell
said.

"Potatoes and beans," Ruby groaned. "I wish it would grow
some pork chops and fried chicken."

"Well, you just sit over yonder in the shade while I load this manure," Russell told her. "It shouldn't take more than an hour or so."

Ruby looked around. Nobody was in sight. Her mama must be in the house and her papa in the back pasture. She watched two bluebirds down the fence row and thought about what she was going to fix for dinner. There wasn't much to fix except the pinto beans and cornbread they had been eating for the last week.

Then she saw it—one of the spring pullets scratching in the dirt on the other side of the lot. It was a white Leghorn and already plumping up with the corn and mash her mama had been feeding it.

Ruby walked toward it saying, "Here, chick, chick, chick," and held her hand like she had some corn in it.

The chicken looked up with its beady eyes and seemed to say, "Well, what do you want? Got something for me?" But it sidled away, still watching her. She wasn't going to be able to catch it without food of some kind. Then she remembered the leftover biscuit she put in her pocket before they left the house. Maybe the pullet was as hungry for a biscuit as she was.

She studied the situation. The chicken was scratching again, but watching her, too. Did she want to give that chicken her biscuit? She could almost taste the blackberry jelly spread between the two halves. But she could taste fried chicken, too.

"Here, chick, chick, chick," she said as she crumbled the biscuit in her hand and squatted on even ground. She spread the crumbs in a trail. "Here, chick, chick, chick," she said again.

The chicken looked at the crumbs, then at Ruby. It was weighing the danger against the smell of the crumbs. It raised one leg as though to step toward Ruby, then thought better of it and stretched its neck as far as it could. But the crumbs were just out of reach.

"Here, chick, chick," Ruby said softly.

The chicken took a tiny step and sort of dillydallied in one spot. Ruby could feel her hands itching to grab that chicken. Then she jumped for it. The chicken skittered away, squawking.

"That dumb chicken," Ruby said, sprawled on all-fours, her stomach dragging on the ground. It took a minute or two to get herself right-side up. When she was on her feet again, she looked over at Russell, but he was still shoveling and whistling. The chicken was pecking again, several feet away.

Then she spied the hook Papa made for catching chickens when her mama wanted one to cook. It was hanging right there on the wall. She backed away toward it and pretended not to notice that the chicken was eyeing the crumbs again.

Then, with the hook in her hand, she squatted several feet away from the chicken. It was now pecking at the crumbs, bobbing its head up and down in obvious delight.

Ruby, behind the chicken, inched closer. She slowly slid the hook along the ground.

Then, fast as she could, she slipped the hook around the pullet's leg and yanked.

She had it! Flapping and squawking in her arms. She hoped Papa wasn't anywhere close around to hear the racket. It was a real scrap, but Ruby managed to grab its neck and clamp its beak shut.

"Ruby, what are you doing with that chicken?" Russell stood over her, his hands on his hips. He looked disgusted.

"I got me some meat. It's just frying size. Wouldn't you like to have fried chicken for dinner?" she asked.

"Ruby, we can't eat your mama's chicken," Russell said.

"Oh, Papa and Mama would like for me to have it if they just knew how hungry I am," Ruby said. She'd detected a little bit of doubt in his voice and played on that.

"Well, you better ask them for it then. It don't set well with me, taking one of their chickens," Russell went on.

Just then, from way on the other side of the pasture, they heard Papa's holler. He looked like a tiny dot heading toward them.

"Let's go," Ruby said as she hoisted the chicken on her hip and held its beak tight. Then she was up in the wagon and pulled the old quilt they used for a seat pad over the chicken to hide it. "I'm having fried chicken for dinner," she told Russell. "You don't have to eat if you don't want to," she said.

Russell must have started to taste that chicken, too, because

59

he jumped up on the seat beside her and clicked his tongue at old Prince who headed out the gate.

Papa caught them just before they turned into the road. "Whatcha in such a hurry about?" he asked.

"We just need to get home with this load of manure, Papa," Ruby said, squeezing the chicken's head as tight as she could. It was squirming, trying to get air. She could feel the quilt fluttering up and down on her lap.

"You feeling okay?" Papa asked her.

"Oh, fine...Papa...fine. I just need to get home and rest," she said.

Russell took off for home, saying, "We'll see you later, Mr. Jim. Giddy-up, Prince."

When they got home, they started right in fixing the chicken. Russell wrung its neck and Ruby put on a pot of water to boil. They made short work of plucking and singeing it.

While it was frying, Ruby began to worry. "I wonder what Mama will think when she counts her chickens."

"Probably think a chicken hawk got it," Russell said.

"It sure smells good, don't it?" Ruby asked. "Do you feel okay about taking it?"

"We've already done it. No use worrying about it now," Russell said. "Make some milk gravy with those drippings."

They sat down and divided the pieces between them. After she had eaten her five pieces and five biscuits, Ruby said, "You know, Russell, I'm glad we saved this chicken from the chicken hawk. I bet Mama would be glad, too."

Walk

by

Paul Milenski

In the nature area behind his house John walked some well-worn
paths, just casually, seeing chipmunks and squirrels, pheasant
and grouse, occasionally a deer. Mr. and Mrs. Collins walked the
same paths. They were quite old, the Collinses, so they walked
slowly in the company of their even-tempered spaniel. When
John saw them coming, he would gear up for a big smile and a polite greeting because the Collinses were fundamentally so amia-
ble. Mr. Collins was president emeritus of a well-established family
company that made paper for paper money. Mrs. Collins came
from a wealthy but hard-luck family. This was her second marriage and it was most clearly not only a very correct marriage, but
a good, loving one. They looked good together, the Collinses—
compatible even in their walking. Then John read in the paper
that Mrs. Collins had died; but maybe it wasn't *the* Mrs. Collins, because after all there were lots of Mrs. Collinses, and maybe it
wasn't her husband who was president emeritus. (John was going
to have to do something about introductions, about remembering names!)

John continued his walks and after a time did see Mr. Collins alone with the dog. Mr. Collins seemed, since last meeting, a

61

little thinner, more gaunt. John and Mr. Collins said hello, stood stiffly facing each other as if in the company of a looming ghost.

"I think you recall that she won't bite," Mr. Collins said, referring to the dog as it moved toward John.

John bent to pet it; its coat was clean and soft and felt like woman's hair. "It's a warm day," John said.

Mr. Collins said, "I thought we would have rain; it's been so humid."

John said, referring to the spaniel, "She's so even-tempered."

Mr. Collins may have smiled amiably. "And how are things going with you; everything is good, I trust?"

John petted the dog. "Yes, it's been a very lucky year. Things are going well."

Then John thought he would say what was on his mind from the first, that he thought it was Mr. Collins' wife's death he'd read about. He wanted to say he was sorry. But he did not know how to say this. Should he say: I am sorry to hear about your tragedy—about your misfortune—about the death of your wife? But what if it were not Mr. Collins' wife? This would be a terrible mistake; it would destroy this meeting, affect today's walk, the quality of future walks. And even if it were *the* Mrs. Collins, then using the terms "tragedy" and "misfortune" seemed inappropriate, as if these terms referred more to fiction than to real life.

John rose, his lips quivering. The dog went back to Mr. Collins. Mr. Collins looked skyward, then to the ground. "This is where you're supposed to be," his look implied. He was talking to her, to his wife, wasn't he?

John finally said, "Have a pleasant walk," and then he felt this was as awkward as saying nothing, as awkward as if he had said he was sorry and subsequently to have been proven wrong—because wasn't it just possible that *the* Mrs. Collins was at home this one time, white work gloves on her frail hands, wiping her hair back from her forehead, instructing and helping the gardener to place annuals here and there? Wouldn't Mr. Collins be pleased when he returned home? Wouldn't he be pleased?

Diggety and the Facts of Life

by

E. Shan Correa

This morning I was whacking away at our hibiscus hedge with
Dad's rusty old pruning shears. One of the problems with living
in Hawaii is that you have to trim stuff all the time because it just
grows back in about five minutes.

I swore at the dull blades when they just folded the branches
instead of cutting them, but I did it kind of quiet because my kid
brother, Jeremy, who just turned six, was right there. He was picking up the trimmings—he called them "bouquets"—and throwing them in the garbage can and talking about Diggety, this dog
in our neighborhood that the Hendersons owned.

"Did you know that Diggety got out again yesterday?" Jeremy
asked. "His grandmother had to chase him all the way down to
the field. Then he stopped to smell a mongoose and she grabbed
his collar."

"*Her* collar, Jer," I corrected. "It's *her* collar and *her* grandmother because Diggety's a girl dog. Boy, it's a good thing you're
going to first grade. You'll learn about gender. Masculine and
feminine. He, she, it and all that stuff."

I started in on the orange bougainvillea. I said, "Put the
gloves on, Jer. These things are full of thorns." For once he
minded me and pulled on our dad's stiff old garden gloves. They

63

went up past his elbows and he looked like a silly robot. The white "Hawaiian Open" cap he had on was too big, too, and when I looked down at him from the ladder, I got this strange feeling, like I had a problem that I didn't even know about before then.

Man! Jeremy doesn't know anything about anything. I mean, he must know that girls and boys are different, and all that, but when he gets to be my age, who the heck is going to tell him about the facts of life?

This probably seems goofy unless you know that my dad died last summer. He'd been sick for a long time, but still his death seemed like a surprise. I was fourteen then, and we'd already had all those man-to-man kinds of talks. In fact, there never seemed to be stuff we couldn't talk about. He knew that he wouldn't be around for long, I think, so he did everything he could to get me ready to help Mom. But I think even Dad couldn't have planned very far ahead for Jeremy.

As I looked down at him I tried to remember Dad's voice. It was deeper than mine. More patient. I tried it out on Jeremy: "Actually, Jeremy, the grandmother isn't Diggety's grandmother, either; she's the Henderson kids' grandmother."

Jeremy wasn't listening. He was getting bored with yard work. He wandered over to the corner of the backyard and found a huge green caterpillar on the lime tree—one of those juicy ones with bulgy blue and green eyes. He watched it crawl up his glove.

"Anyway," he finally said, "Diggety's still getting out."

That was the understatement of the year. Jeremy and I must have helped corral the Hendersons' beagle about a hundred times since they moved here. Like I reminded Jeremy, Diggety's definitely a girl dog, a purebred beagle who's supposed to have purebred beagle puppies. But *she* isn't as choosy about her children's father as the Hendersons are, so she's already had one litter of boxer-beagles and one of some really cute furry black pups that didn't look at all like her.

The Hendersons thought about socking the Tanakas, who own the boxer down the street, with a dog paternity suit, but they didn't. Probably because everybody knows all about Diggety.

64

Diggety's registered name is something fancy, but Mrs. Henderson, who has a neat sense of humor, gave her the nickname and it stuck. She called her Diggety because she was almost always in heat (Diggety, not Mrs. Henderson), which explains why the Hendersons keep her cooped up in the garage so much and also why she always escapes. Jeremy's too young to understand all this, but we always have a few guffaws when we think about "Hot Diggety Dog."

Diggety's suitors howl by the Hendersons' door at night, and in the morning they—the dogs—line up on the lanai waiting for an escape. By then everyone has gone to work or school except the Henderson kids' grandmother, a frail-looking lady who hardly ever comes out of the house except to get the mail and to capture Diggety.

Anyway, when Jeremy and I finished with the trimming, we went back to stuff we usually do on summer mornings. I'd wanted to go boogie-boarding at Sandy's, but most of my friends were seventeen and they were working at McDonald's. I decided to work on my bicycle in the carport. I was putting on my new Shimono neck and polishing the rims, wishing I could show them off to my former girlfriend, Angie; Mom was inside ironing; and Jeremy was playing in the front yard with his cronies, when something happened that was of epic proportions.

"Epic proportions" are two of my new words. All summer I've been devoting myself to two things: increasing my vocabulary and getting over Angie. It's weird, because Angie was the one who helped me the most to get over missing my dad so much, and then, at the beginning of this summer, she dumped me. She said something about me not needing her, and I think she started liking my *former* best friend, Mike, but I really don't understand all of what happened. I know about the facts of life, really, but I don't know if I'll ever understand women.

I wish I could talk to my mom the way I did with Dad, but she's a woman, too, after all, so I only end up getting more and more confused. And lonely. Mom's lonely, too, and I try to help, but when I'm trying to, sometimes I just hear my dad talking in my mind, or see him grinning under his mustache and slamming his big golf hat down on Jeremy's head, and I almost cry, so I just go to my bedroom.

Being the man of the family isn't all it's cracked up to be, believe me. How will I be able to help Jeremy grow up? He needs someone stronger than Mom. He really does.

I shouldn't have said all that stuff. I probably sound like a wimp who just mopes around all the time and that's not me at all. This summer, for instance, I've been using my grief over Angie constructively. I have three vocabulary books and I'm learning twenty-five new words a day so I won't have to express myself with words like "stuff" and "really" and "and so forth" all the time. But now I'm digressing again because I was going to tell you about this morning.

I was in the garage, Mom was ironing inside, and Jeremy and seven or eight other little kids were doing their usual stuff in the front yard. To be more specific, they were pretending they were monkeys in our big tree, teasing about being in love, and bragging about whose dog had rolled over in the most gross stuff— dead geckos, rotten fish at the beach, toad frisbees—you know, the flat dry ones that cars have run over a hundred times—and so forth.

Under the tree were all the kids' dogs. Now every kid in the neighborhood has a dog. There was our old setter. He was a rascal when he was a puppy and that's what his name, Kolohe, means. And there were other dogs with Hawaiian names for "Spot" and "Dog" and "Nose" and stuff. They and their respective kids are always in our yard because we have a Royal Poinciana tree that's the best climbing tree in our whole valley. Really. There are handholds and footholds all over the place and the branches are so strong that only one girl ever broke her arm. She was playing trapeze on the high branches and landed on a big root instead of grass, so her parents knew it was her fault and didn't sue us or anything. So the tree is always adorned with children in it and dogs below.

At any rate, everything was normal when Diggety found a new way to escape from her garage. From where I was working on my bike, I could hear even the top-branch kids, but all of a sudden the noise calmed down, like before a hurricane, and I looked under

66

the old Volkswagen to see why all the quiet. From my gecko's eye view, I could see all the dogs kind of standing at attention.

"Uh, oh. Here comes Diggety!" The cry rang out from the scout with the best view down the dirt road to the Hendersons' place. "Somebody better get his grandmother."

Several pairs of bare feet thudded onto the grass, and one pair hightailed it over to the Hendersons. I stood up just as Diggety pranced directly into the center of the dog population, the white tip of her tail pointing straight at the flowers on the branches above her.

Now, Diggety's the foxiest dog you've ever seen, and her charms weren't wasted, even on old Kolohe. Sometimes when Mom is feeling crazy, she sings *Hard-hearted Hannah, the Vamp of Savannah* for us, and if you can picture Hannah as a dog, that's Diggety. She's gorgeous. Her long ears are light brown and velvety, not all chewed up from fights like our dogs' mangy ears, and her big dark brown eyes are circled by what looks like black mascara or however girls get that look. This is getting embarrassing, so I'll just say that Diggety exudes sex appeal!

Two kids tried to grab Diggety's collar, while two dogs greeted Diggety, their tails wagging a mile a minute. But within thirty seconds it got so noisy my mom came running out the front door.

Man, what a mess! Kids and dogs on every blade of grass, and in a minute they were all out in the street. Dust was flying all over, there were growls and barkings and yelpings and dogs' names being hollered in squeaky voices, and what seemed like a million kids running through the flying hair to get their hands on their own dogs.

"Leave him alone, Jeremy," my mom yelled. "And get out of there. You'll get hurt!"

"Kolohe, come here," someone yelled.

Yelp, yelp…growl, whine….

Around and around everybody went, going so fast it reminded me of that "Little Black Sambo" story where the tigers chased each other so fast they all turned into melted butter. Melted butter. Yes that's exactly what the dogs' blended hairy tan color looked like. They ran in a circle, then they changed course and each one bared his teeth and grabbed another one's tail or ear. It was hard to tell with all the dust, but I thought Kolohe was in the middle.

Yes, Kolohe was there, glomming onto the big lion's mane of a cocker-chow. The chow dog rolled over and just like in judo or something, Kolohe got flipped onto his head. He struggled to get up, all four paws scrambling around in the air, his indignant howl bringing Jeremy into the middle of everything.

"Stop that. You get...out...of there, you stupid dog," Jeremy said as he made a dive for the chow's flea collar and then let out a yelp himself. "Waaaa. He bit me! Kolohe bit me!"

Mom got mobilized even before I did. She streaked over the grass like a mama gazelle, battered her way between the dogs, and zeroed in on Jeremy. Before I was out of the carport, she'd emerged with Jeremy under one arm, and another kid, who weighed at least sixty pounds.

Mom plunked Jeremy and his friend down on the grass and, after checking to see if they were dead or anything, ran back for another rescue. Together we got out Ernest and a little blonde kid I'd never seen before. Then I noticed that the fight was losing momentum.

Diggety, totally unscathed and aloof, had pranced out of the pack. She glanced back toward her house. Sure enough along came the Henderson kids' grandmother, leash in hand. I expected to see Diggety take off full speed when she saw her, but she just danced down the street a little ways, teasing the old lady, who had to gather up the skirt of her long yellow muu-muu each time she lunged toward the beagle.

Meanwhile, Jeremy was still sobbing big coughing sobs, his nose dripping and tears channeling through the dust on his cheeks. Runny noses make my mom feel "noonsch"—a neat Portuguese word that really should be in *Fifty Days to a Zippy Vocabulary* but isn't, probably because they aren't sure how to spell it either—so she started swiping at his face with the Kleenex she always carried in her pocket. I mean *a* Kleenex, not the same one every day, but I'm digressing again...

Kolohe panted over and plopped down on the cool grass beside Jeremy. He licked Jer's arm, all friendly like, and was rewarded by being belted on the back. "Waaaaa...." All the misery that a six-year old's soul could hold was in Jeremy's cry. I could barely make out his words, but it sounded something like "Waaaaa...you stupid dog...gulp...I thought you were my friend...you dummy...waaaa...."

My mom looked at the tiny scratch on the hand that Jeremy extended limply, the same hand that had just punched Kolohe on the back. "You're not hurt, Jeremy," she concluded.

"Yeah, Jeremy. Quit being such a baby." I said it automatically, but as my mom's brown eyes met mine, I was kind of ashamed of myself because I knew that Kolohe was Jeremy's best friend in the entire world, just like Mike used to be mine. So after she gave me that look, Mom gathered Jeremy up in her arms, not even caring about his nose, and patted him until he finally almost stopped jerking and gulping. Then Mom talked to Jer, soft and comforting, and I walked away, wondering what the heck she was telling him.

Because how do you tell a little kid who has problems remembering "he" and "she" about something like Kolohe and Diggety? You really have to be about fifteen and have been through a hell of a lot to understand about sex, and about being betrayed. But whatever she told Jeremy, it seemed to help. Pretty soon he got up off the grass and helped recapture Diggety.

Diggety had decided she didn't really want to leave her fellow dogs and hoof it to the field or to the park. She did some last minute sniffing and socializing and flirting, but she didn't run, so the kids helped hook her leather leash on in record time. But that didn't mean she went along without a protest. No way! She was dragged off by the grandmother, but not in ignominy.

Talk about resisting arrest! Hendersons' grandmother used every muscle, even those flabby ones she must have forgotten about years ago, to pull her down the road. Diggety's legs were all locked at a 45-degree angle forward, and little puffs of dust, like in the cartoons, were left behind each paw as she bounced along. Her neck was all hunched up, and she was still just as stiff and as uncooperative when they turned into the driveway as she'd been when she left our corner. The grandmother looked sweaty, with her nice muu-muu covered with dust and dog-slobber, and I don't remember her coming out for the mail for at least a week.

Jeremy said it all as he watched Diggety's last bounce into the garage: "Diggety...sniff...didn't want...to go back home."

Mom and I looked at each other and started to laugh. We both grasped Jeremy and hugged him and dragged him down on the grass. He didn't know what was going on, but he started giggling, too, happy he'd said something terrifically funny, and all three of us started wrestling and guffawing and rolling around right there in the front yard. The little kids looked at us and each other, then they started in laughing too.

There was my mom lying on her back, flat as a Portuguese man-of-war on the sand at the beach, too weak to lift her hand and wipe the tears off her face, or the grass out of her hair. I tried to sober up, but there was so much fun in her laugh, I just kept starting in laughing again. Mom flung out an arm and leaned it on Jeremy's stomach, and after what seemed like a year, we all got control of ourselves. Then Mom pulled herself up, looked down at us and told us, right in front of all the urchins who were still giggling, that she loved us guys so much.

That was it. Not anything that we didn't know before. I wouldn't even tell about her saying it today except for the way she looked right then, like she'd just rescued the whole *universe* from vicious dogs. She looked strong and full of answers for anything Jeremy or I could ever dream up to ask her.

Wild, huh? It didn't last for long because she remembered she'd left the iron on. We followed her back inside the house. The three of us drank a six-pack of soda and then we finished ruining our lunch by scarfing down a whole box of Twinkies. Then Mom said we'd done a good job on the hedge and the bougainvillea. She promised she'd get the pruning shears sharpened so that from now on, things would be easier.

I remember thinking that things were a little bit easier already.

A Real Bargain

by

Mary Connors

The small red plastic hummingbird feeder tossed on the 25¢ table caught my eye. Tulips, robins, and yard sales—sure signs of spring—were everywhere. This was my first yard sale of the year; it just felt good to have winter done with. I swiftly paid for the feeder, my bargain of the day. *I will commune with nature in peace and harmony...at yard sale prices,* I thought.

When I proudly presented my treasure to Jack, my practical husband, he began asking annoying questions. "Where is the best place to hang this thing? When do you hang it? What kind of food do you put in it? A bargain isn't a bargain if you don't use it. I'm not going to hang the feeder until I can do it right," he said.

Not wishing to display my ignorance, a $5.99 book detailing hummingbird habits seemed like a logical investment. That would protect my 25¢ investment.

The feeder should be hung high, near flowers, in a clearly visible location, sometime early in April, the book read. Armed with this knowledge, Jack surveyed our property for the best site. For several weeks Jack looked. Each morning I would put the feeder next to his coffee cup and finally he could ignore me no longer. "The corner of the balcony is both high and clearly visible," he said. "But Bargain Hunter, there are no flowers nearby!"

71

A $6 investment in petunias and fertilizer solved that problem. Then a $15 half-barrel planter and $5 for planting soil. Now I had furnished the necessary flower bed and another week had gone by.

"To hang the feeder I need an 8-foot length of 1-inch conduit," Jack said. This cost only $6.99. After he finally got started, it really didn't take him long to bend the conduit, fashion an arm on it, drill the hole, attach the hook and then fasten the apparatus to the eaves of the balcony with noncorrosive metal straps. The cost of the straps was a mere $3.95. I consider the two weeks of Jack's spare time and the nagging from me were free.

Hummingbirds feed on sugar water and nectar, the book told me. Sugar, in the height of canning season, costs a paltry $2 for a five-pound bag. The nectar could be purchased at $1.89 for two ounces; with just this one more small investment the "hummers" will be fed and I will be able to watch them while I have my morning coffee.

By the middle of July, only three months later, my "bargain" was ready. The darling little creatures were eagerly anticipated. *Will they forgive the delay? Will sugar water and nectar be appetizing enough or should Kool-Aid be used to lure them? Do they prefer petunias or geraniums?* I nervously wondered. The vision of graciously sipping my morning coffee while basking in nature's tranquility was so close.

Within minutes of the first sugar offering, Ivan the Terrible established his territorial rights. This one-inch red-throated male hummingbird was an absolute tyrant. The fascist decided he was the owner and boss of the feeder. I named him after the meanest dictator I could think of.

Ivan maintained a perch on the clothesline. From there he could guard his feeder when his voracious appetite was appeased. His vigilant perch could be an example for all militia. His watchful head swiveled back and forth anticipating intruders; he protected his treasure. Any audacious hummingbird poaching Ivan's private stock was subject to immediate dive bombing.

Our balcony became a battleground. Zoom!!! Ivan swept down on the trespassers, missing my head by inches. With the precision of a fighter pilot he descended upon his prey and in the process of dodging the little warrior, I soaked my morning paper with spilled coffee. The pugnacious battler drove off groups of two and three invaders of his oasis with fierce determination. Squeaking and chattering, he would strafe bumblebees and wasps. Indeed, if a bald eagle had ventured toward the balcony, Ivan probably would have taken him on.

By mid-September I noticed that Ivan was working overtime. *Migration season,* the book said. Instinct had brought an invasion of Yankee hummingbird travelers heading south for the winter. Our feeder was just a rest stop on their long journey. *Soon Ivan will give up his kingdom, join their ranks and be just another transient,* I mused.

"You have fussed so much about the little varmint I figured you'd be glad to be rid of him," Jack said.

"How dull my morning coffee will be when the little tyrant is gone," I mourned.

The same hummingbirds will return to the same area every spring, the book consoled. And although the 25¢ feeder's final cost was more than $50, didn't I get a bargain!

Concerning Barefoot

by

Mary Connor Ralph

My daughter Lenore's children hang, one from each of her arms, and dangle their milk-pale bodies in the cold Atlantic. Their feet wiggle like small white fish caught in colored nets. Daniel wears blue net swim shoes. Debra wears pink. Her plump toddler's feet keep slipping out; my daughter has misjudged the size of her daughter's feet. Lenore is used to buying shoes with a thumb's length in the toe for growth.

Daniel, clinging to Lenore, eases his feet to the rocky bottom. A large swell reaches us and he squeals, then jumps the wave. "That's my big boy," Lenore says, and he slides from her arm until only their hands connect them.

Foam swirls around us as the waves break. Debra gives me a smile, her face tilted down, eyes looking up at me from beneath the protective brim of her sunbonnet. Her dot of a nose crinkles, cracking the layer of pink sunscreen Lenore has smeared on it. Her delicate fingers push at the sunbonnet, sliding it back to expose wisps of baby-fine brown hair and the beginning of the neat white part Lenore has made by dividing her daughter's hair into two thin ponytails. Without looking at her, as if she senses danger in this tiny restless gesture, Lenore says, "Mother, fix her sunbonnet, would you?"

74

Daniel looks from his mother's face to mine as Lenore and I talk. Lenore asks, "Don't the sharp stones bother your feet?"

Through the shimmering water, our feet wave, side by side, hers slim and long, toes peeking through her white net shoes, the pearl toenail polish making me think of divers on high cliffs above the warm Pacific. My feet are wide, calloused, bulging with blue veins, ending short of hers, the nails yellowed and uneven.

I shake my head and the words escape, "The way you like to trap feet, anyone would think you were the daughter of a fisherman." Daniel's eyes stay on his mother's face, and hers slide sideways to meet them. Lenore doesn't smile.

It's a burden, this waiting for Lenore to be ready to laugh again about her father. I guess it's because she's still young.

It is our first summer here without Phillip. The cottage needs paint, so Donald, Lenore's husband, spends little time on the beach. After breakfast, as I help the children into their swimsuits, Lenore chooses a bottle of sunscreen from her collection and brings it outside where Donald stirs the fresh white paint. Through the window, from the corner of my eye, I see Donald shake his head, see Lenore's pretty mouth curve into a slow pout. When this doesn't work, I hear her voice, "How can you? You know about the ozone. It's not like it used to be. You'll be sick, I just know it."

Donald wipes his hands on his pants, pushes his hat brim back, shakes his head, but takes the plastic bottle from her. Lenore puts her arms around his neck and rests her forehead against his chest.

As we leave the cottage Debra and Daniel turn to wave, "'Bye, Daddy."

"Have fun," Donald calls from the top of the ladder.

I wonder if Lenore sees the unopened bottle of sunscreen jutting from his back pocket.

Mornings, when we walk down the sandy road to this beach, Lenore carries an empty paper bag. She fills it with pieces of broken bottles and sharp bits of eroded metal that might once have been bottle caps. As she bends to pick them up between two slender fingers, she says, "You see, Mother? You see what I mean?"

It strikes me, this is something my mother might have said

75

in summers long past, here in York, where the jagged white beach has always waited down this stretch of sun-warmed road. "Mavis, get something on those feet!" Ma used to call to me.

At the crest of the beach stands a big green trash barrel and, as the four of us reach it, Daniel asks to throw the bag in. Lenore bends down to hand it to him, looks him in the eye, tells him, "You see, Daniel, this is why you and your sister should always wear shoes."

Since she was a little girl, Lenore has loved shoes, but this is something new, some point she has recently reached, a point at which we can never intersect. I have loved barefoot all my life, have never had soft feet, and can't remember a time without callouses and ragged toenails.

When I was seventeen, my girlfriends were going in for open-toed shoes. They were appalled by my feet, the unnatural gray that dusty sidewalks and country roads had dyed them. Sukie Mitchell took to them with a hot soak and pumice stone, and broke the longest of her prized fingernails. Sally Mae Johnson took over, but it was not to be. Finally they packed up their foot parlor and took their fashionable ideas home.

For the Daughters of Deliverance dances, where I was sent to find a suitable young man, Ma forced my feet into white kid pumps. "Soft as newborn skin," she'd say.

"Maybe," I'd tell her, "in *your* hands or on *your* dainty feet."

"Ladies don't complain," she'd say. "It tires men."

When I was twenty-two, and my time for full dance cards was running out, Phillip followed me out from the Mayday Frolic. I felt him watching as I freed my feet from the pumps and stretched my toes into the wet lawn. Inside, when we had danced, his feet hadn't tangled in mine and his hand hadn't strayed from my waist to my hip.

When he stepped from the shadow of the poplars, his scuffed shoes dangled from one hand. He held the other out to me. Inside the music had stopped, but we danced barefoot across the tidy lawns, up and down the streets that circled the Common.

"My barefoot beauty," Phillip called me that summer when we stepped down from the train to honeymoon here in York.

76

On the road where wild roses grow thick as blackberries, I showed him where I used to hide my shoes when I was a child.

The first time Phillip and I set Lenore down barefoot on the Common, she cried. She lifted first one foot, then the other, held her arms out to Phillip, and didn't stop until he scooped her up. Summers, she would walk to the edge of the blanket, then expect to be carried across the hot sand to the water's edge.

When she reached the age of playing dress-up, Lenore was disappointed in me. I had only one pair of dress shoes. Her friends wore a different pair of their mothers' for each new game. They laughed when Lenore wobbled in wearing my old-fashioned black pumps. Ma took her one weekend, to help with the spring cleaning, and she came home with a dozen pairs of Ma's dress shoes, all fit to wear in the company of her friends, all taken from Ma's spare closet.

Now Lenore has a closet in her house just for shoes. Donald built special shelves into it that slide forward so that she can make her daily choices. Even here I've counted six different pairs on her feet in these three days.

Last spring, after we buried Phillip, I came to the cottage one weekend. There was no heat and the sky threatened rain. I walked on the jagged rocks of Lookout Point until my feet bled through the callouses and left dark prints on the granite. I sat in the wind and watched the tide wash the prints away.

Lenore took the train up to search for me and scolded, "Mother, put your shoes on! It's only April. You'll catch your death."

"Your father had shoes on when he caught his," I said. The grieving had made me mean. I wanted to make her cry so we could blow our noses together. I wanted her to take off her shoes that *one* time and walk barefoot with me.

But this was Lenore, after all. The woman who had not cried when Ma died, just because Lenore was as big as a house with Daniel kicking to get born and she had determined that her crying at that stage would upset Daniel, perhaps cause some defect.

For these few weeks this summer I try to bow to Lenore's wish that her children not be encouraged to romp barefoot.

77

Days, I wear stiff sandals or my old tie shoes, my feet bunched into them, tied up like pig's feet in brown butcher's paper.

But evenings are *my* time.

When we've had an early supper of bologna and cheese sandwiches on whole wheat, Donald takes Daniel down to the pier to watch the old men fish. Lenore showers, towels her hair, and picks up her summer romance novel. Her slippered feet rest on the old straw-filled hassock as she leans back in the curved wicker chair on the porch.

Debra's eyes are round as she watches me take off my shoes, uncurl my toes, stretch them. She's still in her bikini, playing with two scarred mussel shells that she dug up on the beach. They're not matching halves, but she fits them together anyway, twisting them gently until the smooth edges almost meet. She holds up this triumph for me to see. "Shells, Grammy."

"Ooh, what pretty shells," I tell her.

She takes them apart, placing one in my abandoned shoe. "Grammy walk?"

"Grammy walk," I repeat.

"Debra walk," she says. Her eyes are ringed with white above her sun-pinked cheeks. Her sunglasses hang from a yellow cord around her neck. She sits on the varnished wooden floor and tugs one tiny sandal. I put my hand over hers. "No," I tell her.

Her mouth quivers. I pick her up, feel her small warmth. She doesn't reach up to hug my neck the way she does in good moments. "Let's ask Mommy then," I say.

I carry her out onto the porch. Lenore looks up. "Walk," Debra says.

Lenore glances at my feet. "I don't know, baby, you still need a bath. It's almost bedtime."

"We won't be long, just a short one tonight," I say.

Lenore's eyes haven't left my feet. I pretend not to notice. "I'm only going to the edge of the marsh."

"Well..." Lenore says.

"Please, please, Mommy," Debra says. It is a small command. Debra knows the right words, but doesn't seem to know she's sup-posed to ask them.

Lenore smiles at her. "Well, I suppose, this once. Just a short one."

I put Debra down, take her delicate fingers in mine. She waves a kiss to her mother and we're off down the gravelled drive to the dirt road. Lenore's voice follows us, "Mother, make sure she keeps her shoes on."

When we reach the edge of the marsh, the sun is going down. Debra holds out her shell, the one she's kept clutched this whole time in her small fist. It's an old shell, pounded smooth by the tides. In the dying sunlight it turns from dull white to pale fire as Debra turns it over and over.

In the salt-water pond, a family of swans paddles toward shore. The babies are a milky necklace between their parents who call to each other as they swim. They've been here for several summers—the same pair, mated for life, raising a new brood each season. Phillip and I discovered them the year he had his first heart attack.

"Look," I say to Debra.

She raises her chin, looks down my pointing finger. A smile takes over her face.

"See? Swans," I tell her. "Big birds."

"And babies," she says.

"And babies," I agree. "Do you want to see their nest?" I ask her.

She nods, making her sunglasses bob on their cord.

The swans disappear behind the tall grass on the edge of the marsh where they've hidden their nest. "We'll have to be quiet," I say. "We don't want to scare them."

Debra sits down in the soft sand, simply dropping to her bottom in that way small children can. She puts a finger to her pursed lips, then bends and tugs her sandals off. She stands, her shell clutched in one hand, her sandals in the other.

I look into her eager face and see this is how it is: we'll sneak up on the swan family, my granddaughter and I. Our bare feet will sink through the white sand until our toes touch that spot beneath the day's warmth, where it's still cool and wet.

Depression Field Hands

by

Dorothy L. Rose

We are a huge crowd of men   women   teenagers
We are people whose cars
Are broken down or
Who have no money to buy gas

Clothed in faded dresses   overalls   straw hats
With sad   dull   listless eyes
We wait hopefully for a day's work
We are at the mercy of the contractor
For transportation to the fields

Mamma has a large ulcer on her leg
Blood-red against her sunburned right shin
An oozing pool of tormented flesh
Festering like the mold on a slab of raw bacon
Just before the Valley heat
Bakes it scabby-black and leather hard

She has to stay off her feet for a while
J T and Imogene stay at the camp with her
They are too young to pick tomatoes

We get up at dawn and walk an hour to get here
Now at 6 AM Daddy and I wait with the mob
For the boss and a truck to arrive at 7
On the corner of Broadway and Main
We pray that we will get work today

Yesterday the truck was loaded
Before we were chosen
If we are lucky today
I will get 5¢ for every crate that I can pick
Daddy will get 10¢ an hour
For stacking and carrying the boxes

Daddy is 43   5'4"   weighs 118 soaking wet
I am 13   small   skinny   towheaded   freckle-faced
Look to be about 11
We are in front of the crowd today

Already the sun glares
From a fierce white sky
Dust swirls on the dirty corner

Last week before our car died
We broke our backs in the tomato fields
The vines made welts on our arms   legs
The sun blistered our faces
Our hands turned a putrid greenish yellow

We made enough money
To pay a week's rent
To buy flour   coffee   lard   beans
But our money has run out again
Mamma's leg is getting worse

We must get work today

I know in Daddy's mind that he is scared
I know what he is thinking
     i wish that i stood 6' tall
     had a little flesh on my bones
     didn't look so hungry
     if they will just choose me
     give me a chance i'll show them
     that i can do twice as much as any man
     just get me on the truck
     i must make enough to get medicine for Mamie
     get her to a doctor
     buy milk for the little ones

And as I swat flies and gnats with my sunbonnet
I stick out my chest
I wait for the truck
I pray that
     the boss doesn't think that I'm too young
     just let me be one of the chosen
     let the job last for weeks
     i want to make enough money
     for more than rent and food
     i want to buy clothes for the family

The truck arrives
Daddy is the last one chosen
There are no more seats
Daddy pleads with the boss
To let me ride in Daddy's lap

As we drive off into the heat wave
I don't look back
I can't stand to look into
The eyes of the crowd

Sale

by

Janis Rizzo

Connie woke up just minutes before the alarm went off. *Today's the day*, she thought, somewhat grateful, somewhat sad.

She slipped out of the half-empty bed and headed for the bathroom. She didn't have much time to get ready, but she'd already chosen her clothes for the day. Her selection had been well thought out, carefully planned: a comfortable pair of beige pants and a yellow and orange flowery, tailored blouse. Bright. Cheery. That would be her mindset for the day, she decided.

The ad had said eight AM, but Connie knew the dealers would be out much earlier, trying to pick through everything first. *Remember: bright and cheery*, she kept reminding herself. After all, these were just things. Lifeless objects. Not values. Not people. Not family.

Family. Her mind started to drift. *We're no longer a family. Twenty-seven long years. Over, just like that*, she thought. She had been so certain she and Ron would always be together. "No," she said out loud. "I won't think about it." She walked to the mirror, stood up tall, and primped her hair.

It was time.

As she opened the garage door, Connie counted five people waiting to descend on their possessions, hers and Ron's. The moment the door was up, they swooped in like vultures, looking and touching. Touching the things they'd shared.

Connie reached down and picked up a hand-painted blue china cup. She passed her hand over the smooth silver ring around the top, then along the dainty handle. It had a large chip on one side. That chip was nearly twenty years old.

She remembered her second child. Henry—then nearly two—had wheedled his way into her lap during a dinner party. As Henry turned to hug his mother, his toy truck smashed into the blue cup, spilling its contents, and cracking the handle. The boy's eyes filled with tears and he buried his head in his mother's shoulder, sobbing inconsolably. Connie had never replaced that cup.

Now, three feet away from her, a young couple was looking over Connie's rocking chair. Ron had bought the beautifully carved maple rocker the day after he found out she was pregnant. He had been thrilled about the news. They had wanted a child so desperately. It had seemed like years till she found out she was expecting.

Connie had settled into the chair immediately and had begun to talk to the baby, Baby Jenny, still seven months away from birth. Every day during her pregnancy, Connie took time to relax in the chair and talk to the baby. And when Jenny arrived, together they spent hours and hours holding each other and whispering their secrets. Then Henry came along and he became the second privileged person to share Connie's chair and her love.

How could this be happening? Connie asked herself, as the young woman sat in the chair and began to rock.

Three months earlier, Connie had been married to Ron. Happily? Well, if not happily, then at least tolerably. They'd had their ups and downs, but they'd managed to stay together—partly for the sake of the children, partly for their wedding commitment, and partly because it was comfortable.

Then, like a bolt from the blue, Ron came home one night and announced he wanted a divorce. Not because of another woman—at least that's what he'd said. Connie *still* didn't understand why. After all, their marriage wasn't so bad; she could have stayed married to him for another twenty-seven years. Why couldn't he?

The more Connie tried to understand, the more angry she became. Then she tried to establish blame. By the time they went to court, Connie and Ron had turned into two hateful, warring factions, wanting to grievously hurt each other. And perhaps wanting to hurt themselves for their own senseless, repugnant behavior.

The day of the hearing, Connie and Ron couldn't even look at each other. Since the life of their marriage and the death of their marriage had taken place in Texas, a community property state, the judge ruled to split everything evenly.

But Connie and Ron could no longer agree on anything, not even on who would get which car. Everything would have to be sold. Everything. The house, the furniture, the cars. Ron's entire workshop. Connie's collection of Hummel figurines. They'd both be walking away with their clothes. And a pile of green paper.

How did things get so out of hand? she wondered now.

Restlessly, Connie walked over to the table next to Ron's radial saw. She stooped over to pick up a white and blue towel, carelessly dropped by a wiry-looking woman who was digging through Connie's neatly folded linens and tossing them aside as if the woman were rooting through trash.

The towel was light blue—both Connie and Ron's favorite color—edged in white Alençon lace, and decorated with white pearls. It had been a wedding gift from her sister Dinah, Connie's maid of honor. Above the lace, Dinah had embroidered Connie's and Ron's names and encircled them with a white heart.

Connie folded the cherished hand towel and placed it back on the table. Then she began to organize the other linens that had been nonchalantly dumped out of the way.

Under the last pillowcase, Connie uncovered a small charcoal drawing of the first home she and Ron had bought. Although never formally trained as an artist, Connie loved to draw, especially outdoor scenes. Her art tended to be simple and honest, very much like herself.

And now she remembered that when the drawing of their small ranch house was completed, Ron had disappeared to his workshop and returned with a simple handmade frame, a perfect complement to her picture. The framed artwork, a product of both their hands, had been granted a place of honor on the wall above their bed.

Connie gazed at the aged sketch, realizing she had been wrong this morning. These were not just things. They were not lifeless objects. They were all remembrances, special mementos with an uncommon life of their own.

As she stood there holding the drawing, a tall man, with salt-and-pepper hair like Ron's, came up to her carrying a square clock radio—the clock radio that had loudly announced that she and Ron needed to begin another day together.

"I'd like to buy this," he said, laying it on the table. "It's marked $5." He reached into his wallet and pulled out a $5 bill. He extended his hand with the money to Connie.

But Connie just stood there, unable to move.

Of Gophers and Boys
at New Year's

by

Jack Boyd

Around Cedar Gap, New Year's used to be the time when boys proved they were almost men (poundwise) and almost gophers (brainwise). That was the time when you took the Christmas gift money you got from non-ambulatory aunts and forgetful uncles and traipsed off to the hardware store to select your New Year's fireworks.

Back in the 1930s, it was a rite of passage for fifth- and sixth-graders returning to school after Christmas to appear with at least one semi-fried thumb and forefinger on one hand.

"Huh," one of the rough boys would smirk, "not smart enough to let go of a live firecracker, are ya?"

"Any sissy can let go," you'd say, holding your shiny, crisp thumb up for group examination. "It takes a real man to let one blow up in his fingers."

"Haw!" the first one would snort. "I got a pocket full a Black Cats right here. We'll go out behind the store shed at recess and we'll just see if you're as brave as you say."

"Black Cats!" you'd say. "My baby sister shoots those off."

The answer would be: "Oh, yeah? I'll bet you burned your

thumb helping your mama cook. You haven't got the guts to hold one of these in your hand."

"You're the one with no guts," you'd argue. "You'd have to hold it with your thumb and finger. I'd hold it with my little fingers."

And the rough boys would boast. "Well, I'd grab it with my whole hand!" one would say.

"I'd sit on it," another would say.

This would be the first plateau, the place for regrouping. The thought of sitting on a live Black Cat firecracker conjured up all sorts of images, none of them truly attractive to the sittee, but of extraordinary interest to the watchers. Second- and third-graders hung back, mouths open and glances darting, sure they were about to witness the bloody end of an entire generation.

Finally came the ultimate challenge.

"Well, if you'll sit on one, I'll sit on one," one of the boys would say.

"Huh! You go first," you'd reply.

One of the third-graders, a snotty-nosed kid sure to wind up a banker, would always say, "Why don't you do it together?" And the only girl interested in burnt offerings would grin and suggest, "And you can light each other's firecracker so neither of you can chicken out."

So, there you were, boxed into bravery by a dare gone sour. There was always a plank and a couple of sticks of stove wood for a makeshift bench. You sat yourself on the plank and took plenty of time placing the firecracker under something solid in your pocket. Otherwise you could wind up with a rosy glow on an extremely sensitive part of your body that would be almighty difficult to explain to a mother or a doctor.

"All right," the girl—it was always the girl!—would finally say, "On three you light the matches, on four you light the fuses."

Everyone backed away as you waited for the wind to die; no sense in having only one firecracker go off because of a dead match. Your heart pounded and your lips went dry as biscuit flour as you remembered your Uncle Toliver's tale of the hired hand who sat on some dynamite and was never exactly right after that.

"One—two—*three*—FOUR!" Both of you fumbled with the lighted matches, banging elbows as you groped for the other's firecracker. Suddenly a sizzling sound would erupt from under your own haunch, and you would slam your match onto the other guy's firecracker and start yelling. Three seconds later the two firecrackers exploded to the sounds of yells and applause. You crow-hopped around and fanned your seat, grinning and trying to think of something profound, or at least funny, to say.

Seen from the vantage point of several decades, the actual explosions were anticlimactic. The denim overalls absorbed most of the noise of the two firecrackers. What was important, however, was the event itself. You had not backed down. You had gone nose-to-nose—or in this case, haunch-to-haunch—with the tough kid from the other side of the hill and you had the scorched hip pocket to show for it.

Actually, you had come out ahead. You had the slick, scaly thumb and finger that the other kid could only envy. You were one up on him, and even better, everybody knew it.

You'd already decided against telling him the truth: that you had scorched your thumb and finger on a pot lid helping your mama with supper.

The Color of Need

by

Susan Rensberger

It was April, the last snow had just melted, the ground was still wet
like a sponge that soaked your shoes when you ran across the
schoolyard. Easter had passed, but our mother was still sick in
bed. She often took to her bed in winter, but that year she was
slower to get up again, and it was especially hard on me. I was
nine years old, my clothes were getting tight, I was starting to
grow up. I needed my mother.

My hair was long then and I had nobody to help me braid it
except for Vera, and she was only in first grade. One morning
when I was walking out to recess, my third grade teacher, Miss
Whitney, put her arm around my shoulders and pulled me aside.

"Would you like me to braid your hair for you, Mavis?" she
asked. I remember her hand on my head, smoothing down strag-
gly wisps. I knew how it looked: my blonde hair looping out
where it was supposed to be close to my head and my braids
crooked because Vera couldn't keep them tight all the way down.
She'd let the hair get too slack and then pull it tight and the
braid would kink. I hated the way I looked, but Daddy wasn't any
use at all with hair.

I couldn't say anything; I was too embarrassed. So I just
leaned against Miss Whitney like a cat looking to be petted and

91

nodded my head against the gathered navy cloth of her skirt. I wondered if she knew Mama was sick and knew what was wrong with her.

I hardly knew myself then, but I knew it had something to do with her mind. And I knew my daddy was tired of it. Nobody had ever told me a name for Mama's sickness. She seemed ashamed of it sometimes, the way she hung her head when you asked her how she was feeling, like you meant it was her fault.

Most times, though, Mama just looked at you like you weren't there, like she could see something nobody else could. Her eyes scared me when they stared like that. I used to think, Why can't she have some respectable sickness, like pneumonia or something? Something the neighbors would bring in food for and we could talk about it in school and everybody would be sorry.

Miss Whitney got a brush from her purse in the bottom drawer of her desk. She pulled a nest of her own dark hair out of the bristles and dropped it in the wastebasket.

I stood still in front of her, better than I ever did for my own mother. I felt proud then, standing at the front of the empty room, the teacher doing my hair for me. I could hear the other kids on the playground yelling to each other, my girlfriends chanting jump-rope rhymes on the sidewalk in front of the school, and the steady *thump-thump* of the tether ball being hit back and forth by eighth-grade girls with strong arms and big fists. But I would rather have been where I was, inside. Recess was nothing compared to having Miss Whitney do my hair.

"You're so blessed, Mavis, with this blonde hair," she said. I could feel my hair twitch and I knew she was untangling the mess Vera had made of my braids. "I've always wanted blonde hair myself." Miss Whitney brushed through it starting at the ends so the tangles wouldn't pull. She was much gentler than Mama.

"Let me see how you look with it down." She had brushed it out smooth all around my shoulders and now she turned me to face her. "Here, take a look." Miss Whitney opened the bottom drawer again and pulled out a hand mirror in a yellow metal frame. I had never seen her use it. I wondered if she looked at it in the morning before we got to school and brushed through her hair with this same brush after she took off her hat.

Miss Whitney was a plain woman, stout, and she must have been around forty then. She had a long nose and little black hairs growing on her arms and upper lip. The hair on her head was black too, with a few strands of gray mixed in, and she wore it short and straight. I tried to imagine her with the long blonde hair I saw around my face in the mirror, but it didn't help her any.

I liked myself better with my hair down that way. I had a round face with freckles and blue eyes like the eyes of a baby doll Vera had that were blue glass and closed when she laid the doll down. I couldn't see anything behind my eyes in the mirror; it was just like looking at the doll.

My teeth stuck out a little in front. My lips were bright red; I always liked them because they gave my face some color. My hair was darker at the top and pale yellow near the ends where the sun had bleached it out the summer before. When it hung down, it covered my ears so they didn't stick out.

"My, aren't you pretty that way?" Miss Whitney said. "When you're older and your parents let you do your own hair, you might want to wear it down like that."

"I do my own hair now, except Vera has to help 'cause I can't braid the back and Mama's sick. I braid Vera's for her, only I do it better 'cause I'm older," I said.

"I'm sure you do. You're such a good helper. Your mother's lucky to have a daughter like you," Miss Whitney said. "I'm sorry to hear she's not feeling well. It must be hard for you and Vera."

"Sort of," I nodded. "Mama does get up to fix supper, most times. Vera and me can fix our own lunches and Daddy does the wash. He doesn't like to fold though, so Vera and I do that. But none of us can iron." I smoothed down the wrinkled skirt of my dress while I talked. I'd forgotten how it must have looked.

"Well, maybe we can find someone to come in and do the ironing while your mother is sick," Miss Whitney said. "Don't you worry, an ironed dress isn't near as important as a sharp mind." She finished my hair while she talked, put the rubber bands back on the ends of my braids and showed me the mirror again.

She had parted my hair on the side instead of down the middle like I usually did and it looked special. I liked my new image much better than the way I'd looked in the bathroom mirror that morning before I left for school. Miss Whitney gave me a long hug when I handed the mirror back to her. I leaned against her and she held me tight.

"Your mother is really blessed to have her own little girl and to have it be you," she said. I felt so still inside, like I had to hold my breath not to spoil anything. When I remember that time now, the school room looks different than it did other times, like looking at it through a colored window. Only I can't name the color; it's the color of need, I suppose.

The school bell rang and made us both jump. Miss Whitney let go of me and put her brush away. My friend, Ilene, noticed my hair right away and asked if that's why I stayed in at recess. I said yes, and all my girlfriends thought I was lucky to have Miss Whitney do my hair. I was just glad they thought it was something special instead of making fun of me for it. I could never tell which way those things would go, those things that made me different.

That afternoon I remember walking into the house with Vera. We stood still in the back hall, listening. Our daddy's truck wasn't in the yard. That meant he was out someplace. We listened to see what Mama was doing. Every day we hoped she might be up fixing supper. Sometimes she was, and she might be dressed and combed or she might be in her pink chenille bathrobe with her hair hanging down and tangled, shuffling around the kitchen, doing her duty, but not really there.

One day she'd get up out of bed and stay up, tuck us in at night and then be up before us in the morning cooking us oatmeal. We kept believing that day would come again, like it had before, though she'd never stayed sick in bed as long as she did this time. That day we listened and we didn't hear anything, not her shoes clicking on the linoleum or slippers shuffling or even crying from the back bedroom. Nothing to tell us she was there.

We took off our coats and went on tiptoe through the house, back to the bedroom where Mama slept when she was sick and not sleeping upstairs with Daddy. She had the shades all

94

down and the room was dark. It smelled warm and sleepy and close, like my pillow when I woke up in the morning before I lifted my head. Her bed was pushed up against the far wall and she was turned away from us, lying on her side curled up in a ball. She might have been sleeping or just lying there with her eyes closed. She could do that for hours. Vera tiptoed back out like we usually did and went to the kitchen to look for a snack.

But I stood there, looking at my mother's tangled hair on her pillow. I went over to the east window and put the shade up just a little, so I could see. Then I went to the bathroom and got the hairbrush out of the cupboard and went back and sat down beside Mama, and started brushing her hair.

It wasn't as long as mine and Vera's—she'd cut some of it off—but it still hung below her shoulders. I picked up a handful that had wound around itself and began brushing it out, starting at the bottom like Miss Whitney had done and working back up, holding the hair tight above the tangles so when I had to tug, it wouldn't pull the roots. Mama's hair was soft brown, that medium-dark color like Vera's. It had some gray in it, a little more than Miss Whitney's, although my mother was younger.

When I'd gotten the tangles out I began brushing gently from the top down. I was careful not to knock the brush against her head. I brushed the side and then the back, my free hand following the brush, smoothing down the hair. I brushed my dog Willie that way sometimes, petting him so that he'd hold still.

"That feels good," Mama said finally. Her voice was so small and quiet I could hardly hear. It sounded hoarse, creaky like when you first get up in the morning. I wondered when she'd last said anything.

"Sit up, I'll brush the other side," I said. She sat up just like I told her and turned around. She sat cross-legged in her long white nightgown and looked at the wall over the head of the bed while I got up on my knees and brushed the rest of her hair.

"Do you want me to braid it?" I asked.

She looked at me finally then and smiled, just the littlest smile but the first one I'd seen in a long time. I wondered if her

95

mouth felt stiff. Her eyes looked sad, but at least I knew they were looking at me.

"No thanks, honey. Maybe I'll just leave it down awhile; it feels so good now you've brushed it." She hugged me and I squeezed her back. Then she pulled away from me and looked again. "Your hair looks real nice. Who parted it that way for you?"

"Miss Whitney braided it for me," I said, "'cause Vera didn't do it tight enough and it was all coming down."

My mother didn't say anything, just looked back at the wall. I remember how scared I felt then, afraid I was going to lose her again. I wish I hadn't mentioned Miss Whitney, I thought. *It might make Mama feel like I liked Miss Whitney better.*

"I'm so glad you're my mama," I said. I hugged her as hard as I could, put my head against her chest and was sorry for all the times it wasn't true. I did want her for my mama, but I wanted her to be well.

"Should I brush your hair every day like that?" I asked. I was trying to get her to look at me again. She did. She looked back down at me and stroked her hand up and down my back like she used to when she tucked me in at night.

"You don't have to take care of me, honey," she told me.

"I'm just brushing your hair. It feels so nice," I said.

Mama didn't say anything for a moment, then she answered in her slow voice, like she was thinking through every word. "Yes, it does. It feels good to have somebody take care of you, doesn't it?"

She held me a long time, rocking me on her bed till after a while I knew she wasn't doing it for me anymore, but for herself. I had an old stuffed bear I used to hold like that sometimes, so I knew how she was feeling. I curled up on her lap as small as I could and let her rock me.

Finally we heard the back door open and Daddy's step in the hall. Mama looked guilty and let me go.

"Goodness," she said, "it's time for supper, isn't it?"

I always believed that was the day she started getting better. Now, of course, I know it wasn't as much my doing as I thought at the time. She always did get better in the spring; sooner or later she'd have gotten out of bed anyway. Still, I think I did help her.

Every day after school, for the rest of April and on into May, until after the trees had sprouted their leaves, I'd brush her hair until she noticed me. I believed I had the power in my own hands to reach her, the way Miss Whitney had reached me, the power to make her better.

One day when Vera and I got home from school, Mama was up out of bed. She'd done her own hair and gotten dressed and she was in the kitchen starting supper. For a long time after that she was good and she took care of us.

But I kind of watched. Now and then, when I thought she seemed a little low, I'd go get the hairbrush and ask could I brush her hair. "Sure, honey, if you want to," she'd say. And I'd sit beside Mama and brush out the tangles, keeping her with me as long as I could.

Rexie-Boy Reinhardt

by

John Buchholz

The little village slept in the intense afternoon heat and my bent bicycle pedal clanked monotonously against the kickstand as my Schwinn and I, the only animate objects on Elm Street, would zig-zag from house to house along our daily route.

Whistling "Zip-A-Dee-Doo-Dah," I bounced over Snyder's front yard and winged a folded *Times-Union* behind my back toward their front door. Clearing the delicate Victorian railing and sailing neatly between the pillars, the paper slapped the shiny gray porch floor and skidded to a stop under Mrs. Snyder's rocking chair.

"B-plus," I told myself.

As I peddled toward Jensen's porch, plotting another tricky shot, a subtle movement off in the distance caught my attention. Curious, I stopped my bike, shaded my eyes and squinted far down the hot slate sidewalk.

My curiosity suddenly turned to terror. The tiny black cannonball hurtling toward me through the undulating heat waves was none other than Rexie-Boy Reinhardt, the fiercest dog in town.

Since the day I took over the route, Mrs. Reinhardt, who was my fourth-grade teacher, had insisted that Rexie-Boy learn to retrieve the newspaper from my hand and carry it home. She smiled from behind the screen door as the beast curled its upper lip, exposing teeth that looked like railroad spikes. "We'll start," she said, "with you pushing it through the mail slot to him for a few days." She turned toward the snarling animal. "Paper, Rexie-Boy! Paper!"

He attacked it as I poked it through, then dropped the soggy, shredded mess at her feet. "Good boy!" she exclaimed, patting his square head. "Rexie-Boy is Mommy's sweet lover-boy!"

"I don't think he likes me very much, Mrs. Reinhardt," I said.

"Nonsense!" she replied. "Don't be afraid of him. He'll never bite you. He's just a big actor. Next week we'll train him on a leash in the yard."

A few days later, they met me on the lawn. Rexie-Boy's short black hair bristled, his evil red eyes burned at me, and he growled like an idling motorcycle as I cautiously approached with the folded *Times-Union.*

"Give it to him! Give it to him! Paper, Rexie-Boy! Paper!" Mrs. Reinhardt shouted, holding the taut leash with both hands as he lunged, snatched it from me, and tore it to pieces. "Oh, Rexie-Boy is Mommy's best little sweetness!" she gushed, wresting the mangled paper from him as I beat a hasty retreat to my Schwinn.

Straining at the leash, the brute bared his teeth and Mrs. Reinhardt smiled broadly. "You know," she said, "one of these days, he'll meet you down the street and bring it home all by himself!"

"Mrs. Reinhardt," I protested, "I'm not sure that's a good idea. I don't think he likes me very much."

"Of course he does," she insisted. "Growling is just his way of saying hello. He does it to the mailman, too." With that she dragged Rexie-Boy toward the house, a low snarl burbling deep in his throat. As the screen door banged behind them, she turned and proclaimed, "All by himself one of these days!"

Now my biggest fear had come true. The crazed canine's studded collar glinted in the sun and his feet did not seem to touch the sidewalk as he thundered toward me. Gripped with terror, having no place to run and only seconds to act, I quickly folded a newspaper, maneuvered my trusty Schwinn across the walk and crouched behind it. Then, like a matador baiting a charging bull,

I dangled the *Times-Union* on his side of the rear fender. "Mommy's best little sweetness!" I screamed. "Paper! Paper!"

He was flying low, and although it was patently clear it wasn't the paper he was after, I fired it at him anyway. It rocketed past his head and skidded down the sidewalk, but the raging mass of bone and muscle was undeterred. Misjudging his speed, he shot by me, braking in a cloud of dust immediately to my rear. I made a desperate move toward the other side of my bike, but it was too late. He pulled a quick U-turn and leaped.

I watched in horror as his long ivory fangs plunged through my new chinos and deep into my calf. He gurgled in ecstasy and tugged at my leg as I vainly beat his iron head with my fist.

Then it was over. Satiated, he unclamped my leg, gagged, coughed, and turned toward home, trotting nonchalantly past the newspaper. I hurled a string of uncomplimentary epithets at him, but he was unfazed.

Warm blood oozed down my leg and my white sock turned sticky dark red as I clanked five blocks to Dr. Wood's office.

"Grit your teeth," he warned, cauterizing my wound with a long cotton swab soaked in hydrochloric acid. "This'll burn some, but you'll be okay." Tiny wisps of smoke curled up, and I watched my pink flesh cook and turn gray. "I'll notify Mrs. Reinhardt," he said, taping a gauze compress over my new black stitches.

Later, after I finished my route, Mrs. Reinhardt called to apologize. "Don't worry," she assured my mother, "Dr. Wood will send me all the bills, and I'll keep that naughty little Rexie-Boy in the house until he learns to behave and says he's sorry!"

Contrition, however, was never to be a part of his antisocial personality. Each time I rode by during his incarceration, wary of an ambush, I would fling the folded *Times-Union* all the way from the front sidewalk to the welcome mat, and Rexie-Boy would hurl himself against the screen door.

Nevertheless, after a week had passed, convinced that he had learned his lesson, Mrs. Reinhardt released him one sleepy afternoon just as the mailman sauntered around the corner.

Dr. Wood did his stitches, too. And after that day, no one ever saw Rexie-Boy again.

Surviving with Sorghum

by

Lee Hill-Nelson

Long hot summer days called for mischief on the farm in rural Texas. At mid-afternoon three hungry, barefooted girls stood in a circle watching Bud, our brother, stir sorghum syrup candy. The thin brown liquid rolled and boiled in a black-iron skillet on an antique kerosene stove.

Sorghum grew in our area, and with a syrup mill nearby, it was inexpensive. The syrup (pronounced "serp" in Texas) was thick, dark, and sweet. Mixed with cow's butter on flapjacks, the syrup was quite tasty. With peanut butter, it made a filling meal. The empty syrup buckets were the right size for school lunches and the right size to set under a cow for milking.

"Keep back, you kids. You'all gonna get burned," Bud yelled as we strained forward to see the progress of the treat made from sorghum syrup, water, sugar, and vanilla flavoring. Then we heard soft footsteps coming down the hall. Mama was up from her nap!

The year was 1932 and we were in the Great Depression. Because sorghum syrup had a long shelf life, it was a main food item in our home. Candy-making was forbidden, but we sometimes broke the rules.

As Mama's footsteps neared, Bud knew he was in big trouble. He grabbed the skillet and ran through the back door into the path of a setting hen who was a vicious creature. She was angry and flew at Bud's bare feet and pecked them with her sharp bill. Just as he outran the hen, the loose skillet handle turned and the red hot candy hit his feet.

Poor Bud! His feet were hurting from the hen pecking and the candy burning, and there was no candy left to eat. He got a scolding, but that was not the last time he cooked sorghum syrup candy.

The very next day, Bud brazenly made another batch and there were plenty more times after that Bud made the verboten treat behind Mama's back. But he never came away empty-handed again.

Before Bud died last year, he often told his children and grandchildren the story of the setting hen. He promised to make them some syrup candy, but he never did.

When I see sorghum on the store counters, I wonder if it really tastes the way I remember. I sometimes think I will buy some and make some candy, but then I don't want to spoil the memory of the candy Bud had made.

Goodbye Venice

by

Jim Adams

"No!" Elaine's voice was loud in the examination room, causing echoes. "I won't allow it." She scooped up the cat, a white Angora with a lackluster tail, from the counter and hugged it close.

"I'm sorry," said the veterinarian, startled by Elaine's vehemence, "but simple old age is beyond my..." His voice trailed off as he groped for the words to mollify the short, fiftyish, slightly plump woman that stood before him with a stubborn expression on her face, her lower lip trembling. Elaine's usually good-natured features were familiar to him; she had brought the cat to see him every few months since her husband died, at least eight, perhaps ten, years ago.

Uncertain of her own next move, poised for possible fight or flight, Elaine stood shifting her weight from one foot to the other, her stylishly trimmed, brown-with-gray-streaked hair quivering slightly at the tips.

The vet began again. "Felinity has had a long, good life, but the time has come when it would be a kindness..."

"No," Elaine repeated, more quietly, cupping a hand over the cat's ears as though protecting her from unpleasant news. Felinity's eyes—one amber, the other pale blue—were half shut. In some spots the cat was semi-bald with pink skin showing through the fur. Hundreds of cat hairs clung to the front of Elaine's tweed skirt and jacket.

The vet removed the stethoscope from around his neck and dropped it into the pocket of his lab coat. "Sometimes," he said, speaking with elaborate patience, "when we're lonely, we get so involved with our pets…"

"I'm taking her home," Elaine interrupted. She whirled and, almost running, left the office to find a taxi.

At home, a brown brick townhouse, Elaine tucked Felinity into her satin-lined cat basket and switched on the heating pad under the pillow. All evening she pampered the cat, cuddling it and grooming it gently with her favorite brush. She sautéed a chicken liver in butter, but Felinity refused to taste it. Then she cut out and stitched together a flannel mouse and filled it with imported French catnip, but Felinity couldn't be roused to notice, let alone play with it. Soon hot tears, unwelcome guests, dropped in and stayed the night.

In the morning, following a slow, cold, gray November dawn, Elaine carried Felinity back to the pet clinic and left her there.

That afternoon she phoned a travel agent, picked at random from the Yellow Pages, and ordered a ticket to the first destination the agent mentioned. Venice, as it happened.

Ignoring the intermittent rain showers that damped the evening, Elaine pushed her way through a cluster of tour groups—French, German, Japanese—being lectured in several languages at once in the Campo San Bartolomeo. Squeezing between the wheels of gaily decorated snack carts pushed close against the tourists by shouting vendors, she edged her way past the church's granite steps to the Riva del Ferro.

Gamely pursuing art, culture, and romance, she entered any building open to the public, guidebook in hand. Art and culture she found in plenty in the palazzi, the churches and the museums. Romance, though, proved just as elusive in Venice as it was at home. Even the legendary ardor of Latin Lotharios seemed to have been exaggerated: in the past week, Elaine's thighs hadn't been pinched even once.

Out on the street, a cat, one of the countless felines that roamed the byways of the ancient city, reached up and snagged the hem of her new raincoat. Elaine paused and, for the hundredth time that day, pulled a tidbit of mozzarella from a plastic bag tucked into her purse. The cat, black with tan splotches, ignored the proffered cheese and ran a few steps into a narrow lane separating time-worn brick buildings that smelled of mold and rotted seaweed. There it stopped and gazed back at her with crystal green eyes, impatiently twitching its tail.

Elaine walked softly toward it, her hand extended. "Here, kitty," she called.

Again the cat ran as she approached, but it soon paused, glancing back impatiently as though to say, "Hurry up, won't you?"

Elaine followed until she saw the boy, dressed only in a pair of baggy cotton trousers, huddled against a crumbling wall. His head rested heavily on his knees. His thin, bare shoulders shook with sobs. Elaine's guidebook offered no Italian phrases to fit this situation.

Feeling helpless in the face of his obvious misery, she groped around in her Gucci shopping bag till she found an orange. She touched his shoulder and offered it to him. With a startled look of gratitude he accepted it and stuffed it into his pants pockets. He jumped up and, bowing low, kissed the hem of her raincoat. Elaine blushed with embarrassment. Barefoot and dirty-faced, the boy might have been eight or nine.

The black-and-tan cat had disappeared. Elaine backtracked to the Riva del Ferro, her feet and legs sore from a day of slogging over cold, wet paving stones in thin-soled shoes.

"Meow-r-r-r!" A calico street cat yowled up at her, begging for a handout.

"Are you speaking Kitalian?" Elaine asked it. She offered it the last bit of mozzarella, but the calico, apparently better fed than its cousins, only sniffed at it and drew back as if saying, "Not good enough." It trotted away, tail indignant, to panhandle diners seated beneath red-and-white striped Cinzano umbrellas at an open- air café. Elaine shrugged and set off again. A few steps down the street, a hand tugged sharply at the back of her raincoat. Frightened, Elaine whirled about and lifted a defensive arm.

"Oh. It's you," she said. She stared down at the boy, at his eager eyes half hidden by tangled, black hair. He seemed oblivious to the drops of rain trickling on his olive skin as he held out to Elaine the reluctant calico that had spurned her cheese. "How sweet," she told him as she stroked the cat's fur. She opened her purse to dig for loose change.

"You! American *signora!*" a policeman shouted from across the street, his black mustachio fierce with disapproval. "Give him nothing. Begging is not permitted."

Elaine flushed and snapped her purse shut. "No *lira,*" she told the boy, vigorously shaking her head and shooing him away.

The boy wilted. He dropped the cat and darted away into the forest of legs that pulsed along the pavement.

Elaine resumed her push toward the worn marble steps of the Rialto Bridge. Festively decorated with thousands of tiny white lights, the bridge glittered above the evening mists rising from the Grand Canal. An odd feeling of being watched caused Elaine to glance back over her shoulder as she climbed. The boy was following her, lurking from doorway to shadowy doorway, staying a few paces behind. She caught his eye and gave him a solid glare, until he turned around and shuffled away.

A mosquito whined past, chased by a squall blowing in from the Adriatic. Elaine's hair whipped wetly around her cheeks and ears. In the middle of the bridge she stopped abruptly and leaned against the balustrade, just above the marble dove. Caught by a wave of homesickness, she stood stroking the cold stone with uncertain hands, gazing with unseeing eyes at the speedboats and *vaporetti* plying the choppy, gray-green water of the canal.

From the arch beneath her feet slid a black gondola, poled by a boatman flinging an aria into the teeth of the wind. Two lovers, entwined on the plush gold passenger couch, kissed passionately, oblivious to the rain.

Elaine pulled a tissue from her bag and dabbed away raindrops and tears. City of romance, my foot, she thought with some bitterness. Last night, wearing a new—and criminally expensive—green cocktail dress cut low enough in front to display an almost indecent amount of cleavage, she had stayed until near closing time in Harry's Bar.

Growing tipsy on Bellinis—the house drink of fresh peach juice and champagne—she had patiently warmed the seat of a wooden chair the bartender assured her was Papa's own. But, other than offering polite acknowledgments of her presence, none of the men tried very hard to engage Elaine in a serious conversation or offered to buy her a drink. She had left in a huff when she overheard—or at least thought she overheard—a comment about "ugly enough to make a Venetian blind."

A pigeon fluttered to the railing and, balancing precariously against the wind that fanned its tail feathers, pecked its way toward Elaine's fingers. "No fool like an old fool," she informed it.

Bigger drops of rain splashed. To hell with men, Italian or otherwise, Elaine decided. Anyway, tomorrow I have to go home. She descended the steps on the far side of the bridge and took a shortcut through the back streets toward her hotel, looking forward to a hot bath, the latest edition of *L'Espresso*, and the pound of Viennese chocolates stashed in her shopping bag. Perquisites of the lonely, she told herself.

Below a shop window displaying Murano glassware—a set of sapphire blue goblets and a school of aquamarine fish with crystal fins revolving on mirrored trays—crouched a white kitten, soaked and miserable.

Wanting to help, Elaine reached to pick it up, but it hissed and, quick as a ferret, clawed her and ran. "Damn!" she said, irritated with herself for being so incautious.

She licked at the scratch on her thumb and peered anxiously into the swirling fog. Full darkness shrouded the city and the deserted back streets were filled with small, nervous sounds—wavelets lapping at foundation stones, tiny squeals from boats rubbing against their mooring poles, the hiss and gurgle of drain spouts emptying into catch basins.

From the top of a wall, a row of terra-cotta gargoyles leered at Elaine with fanged, evil mouths. Her pumps whispered more quickly on the paving stones. Slick with rain, the stones gleamed where an occasional light cut into the gloom.

Close behind Elaine, a foot splashed. Pulse hammering, she whirled to look. A short, familiar figure crept closer, gripping the white kitten.

What does he want, she wondered, a thrill of fear shooting through her. "Go away," she tried to shout, but the sound caught in her throat and emerged as little more than a whisper. She hastened across a footbridge spanning an inky canal and ran clumsily, the tails of her raincoat fluttering like pigeon wings.

The boy ran too, racing on bare feet, gaining on her, shouting, "Hey! Hey!"

Completely unnerved, Elaine rushed into the Hotel Bellini and up the carpeted stairs to her room. Gasping for breath, she slammed the door and bolted it and dropped onto the bed. When her heartbeat slowed and air flowed smoothly into her lungs again, she undressed and crawled between the sheets, soothed by the tap dance of wind-driven raindrops on antique leaded panes.

Elaine awoke refreshed, pleased to see bright, unexpected rays of sunshine highlighting the baroque red and gold carpet. She quickly showered and, slipping into a lightweight, navy blue dress for her last day in Venice, stepped out on her diminutive balcony to brush her hair.

All the clouds and fog had blown away. The sun beat down on gray stone churches, red brick towers, and legions of orange-tiled rooftops. Breezes carried tidal smells from the lagoon, flat and blue in the distance. Socks and underwear fluttered like giddy sea birds on clothes lines strung between houses. From the people thronging the constricted lanes below rose hearty shouts and easy laughter.

At the hotel doorway, Elaine's good mood was quickly jarred. The boy sat waiting on the stoop, though he hadn't spotted her yet because he was watching a red-spoked flower cart being pushed past. Elaine clenched her fingers into frustrated fists. "Go away or I'll call the police—the *Polizia*," she shouted.

He didn't turn.

"Go away!" she repeated.

Still no response.

She moved close behind him, wondering, "You! Young man!" she said loudly, her voice shrill. He didn't stir so she gave up, shaking her head, and stepped past him into the street.

"Hey!" he shouted as soon as he saw her. He jumped up and, eyes pleading, held out to her the white kitten.

Elaine paused, a hesitant knowledge growing in her, finally reaching certainty.

He's no beggar, she realized with a shock, he's *deaf.*

Her cheeks burned when she remembered her fear, her running from him. She forced herself to relax and accept the kitten, snuggling it to her breast where it purred contentedly.

Elaine smiled warmly at the boy and he grinned back, his crooked teeth milky against his dusky cheeks. "Hey," he muttered, thrusting his hands deep into his pockets and squirming his toes.

Elaine put the kitten down. It climbed into a planter box gay with yellow jonquils and curled up for a nap. Elaine flared her fingers and motioned with both hands toward the boy to wait. She hurried back upstairs to her room and dug the Trailblazers T-shirt out of a suitcase. Okay, he's a little short, she thought wryly, but at least I get to give it to a friendly male.

The T-shirt fit the child like a sack, but looked fine once he tucked its tails into his trousers. Elaine pointed to her camera. The boy stood straight and smiled, a proud look on his face. Elaine snapped a picture and waved goodbye. She went back into the hotel and left it again through the rear exit.

She spent several hours in St. Mark's, wandering past the gruesome displays of martyr bones, the stained glass, the golden altars, the jeweled relics stolen from around the world. She bought packets of corn and fed the flocks of parti-colored pigeons that followed her around the piazza outside. Though she had no romantic encounters, discounting the 100,000 *lira* brazenly offered by a squat Egyptian businessman in a red fez, she had fun. She even began to think that Venice might, when the sun was shining, really be a city of romance.

"Hey!" The shout rang out behind her when she paused in a sun-washed piazza near the Grand Canal to buy an orange soda. A squadron of pigeons, startled by the noise, launched themselves into the air for the obligatory once-around-the-fountain and settled down again.

The boy came running, still wearing the T-shirt, carrying a tatty brown cat with frazzled ears. He held it for Elaine while she petted it, his eyes worshipping her face. He released the struggling animal and ran to grab up another, an orange-and-white-spotted tom from under a wooden-wheeled pastry cart.

He must know every cat in town, Elaine thought. I suppose I'll have to pet them all.

To distract him, she led the way into a Chinese café and ordered sweet and sour prawns. "Whoa," she said with mock severity, snatching the soon empty serving platter from him. "We don't lick plates in public."

He grinned and carefully licked his fingers instead, then wiped them on the tablecloth.

Back outside, the afternoon shadows had lengthened considerably. "I have to go away. On a plane," Elaine told the boy, pointing to herself and making her hands swoop like an airplane.

If he understood, he didn't show it. He grabbed a fold of her dress and insistently tugged her toward a narrow catwalk hidden between a rococo church and a villa whose walls were a patchwork of cracked and flaking plaster.

"All right." She sighed and allowed him to guide her though she was very aware of the time and her need to pack up her luggage. She followed him through the dank passage, careful not to brush her dress against the grimy walls. The boy led her under a low arch guarded by two weather-beaten stone lions and a skewed, rusty gate.

They stood in a walled garden overrun with weeds and flowering vines, shaded by trees whose unpruned branches tangled together above their heads. Perched on the cracked marble lip of a dripping pedestal fountain, a tabby dangled its claws in the water trying to hook a goldfish. The boy seemed vastly pleased when Elaine looked admiringly around at the white and yellow daisies growing in profusion.

On a bench carved from limestone they rested companionably in the dappled shade until Elaine heard, in the distance, the bronze Moors atop the clock tower strike the bell four times with their iron hammers. She stood up in haste and sadly shook the boy's hand. "I'll miss you," she told him, setting off quickly toward the gate.

"Hey!" the boy yelled before she had gone five steps. Elaine turned and saw him lift his fingers to his lips. Looking directly at her, an unreadable expression on his face, he blew a piercing whistle that echoed off the garden walls. From under the shrubbery, yawning and stretching, emerged several cats. A dozen more dropped from tree branches and trotted purposefully toward Elaine with their tails curled into fishhooks.

Elaine moved to leave, but a rabble of cats stormed through the gate and blocked her path. She froze, surrounded by cats. Paunchy cats, striped cats, frizzy cats, all with feral, sharp-featured faces. Hissing and growling and shouldering each other aside, they swarmed about her, rubbing their whiskery cheeks on her nervous calves. When she tried to wade free, a score of paws grabbed at her ankles, keeping her off balance. Her nylons ran in a dozen places where exploring claws hooked into the delicate fabric.

The caterwauling grew louder and more cats appeared atop the garden wall, leaping down to the grass and running to join the unruly mob. Elaine's face paled. A half-grown kitten leaped onto her dress and began to climb, needling its claws into her thighs until she was forced to slap it off. She grew dizzy and claustrophobic, trapped in a heaving sea of fur and tails and glittering eyes.

All at once, leaving Elaine gasping for breath, the cats deserted her, running toward an iron-banded door in the garden wall that was screeching open on rusty hinges. Through the door rolled a loaded cart, pushed unsteadily by a surly crone. A ciga-

111

rette hung smoking from a corner of her mouth, dripping ashes onto her long, black dress. Releasing the cart handle, the old woman waved a gnarled hand toward the boy and disappeared, thunderously slamming the door.

A hundred cats, some up on their hind legs, danced in a frenzy as the boy pushed in among them to distribute cans of pungent meat and reeking fish parts. The cats snarled and clowned, knocking over the cans and boxing each other for choice tidbits.

Now that she knew why the cats swarmed so, Elaine lost her fear and pushed in to help, lifting double handfuls of sardines from the cart and tossing them to cats that caught them on the fly. When the food was gone, the cats, one by one, disappeared into the bushes or trotted out the gate with smelly prizes locked in their jaws until only a few remained, rolling contentedly on the sun-baked paving stones.

Elaine and the boy washed their hands in the fountain. She rubbed a spot of dirt from his cheek with motherly fingers and smoothed his hair. "You're full of surprises," she said. He gazed up at her, an adoring look on his face.

"I'll say it for you," Elaine told him. "I'm beautiful. Thank you. No one has thought so for a long, long time."

Caught short by a surge of raw emotion, she backed away, her heart pounding. She gestured to the boy to stay and determinedly strode off. At the gate she paused, sensing his gaze. *I have to go home,* she told herself. *I'll miss my plane.* But still…

She turned to look at him once more.

"Oh, come along, then!" Elaine said. She beckoned and the boy raced across the grass to her, his white teeth and happy eyes flashing with excitement. "Let's go find out who you are," she told him.

Hand in hand, they left the garden to the cats, who, being cats, just yawned and pretended a vast indifference.

Salmon and Bullheads

by

Lucille Bellucci

Millie and I have been married thirty-nine years, not as long as some couples, but a lot longer than many. We know each other pretty well.

Of course she could tell how I was feeling when I came back from my fishing trip up the delta, east of San Francisco.

"Sit down and get warm first," she said. "Never mind taking off your boots, just yet. Here's some hot soup I made this morning. I put chunks of marrow in it, the way you like it."

I looked at my wife's sympathetic face, a little rounder than it used to be, and puffy in the mornings when she got up, but none of that changed the fact that I loved her. For some reason she loved me, too, though you wouldn't know it from the way she often got exasperated with me. When I retired two years ago, there were a shaky couple of months when I thought she was about to run out and look for a job just to get away from me.

The soup tasted wonderful. I began to relax. "The whole Bay isn't what it used to be, never mind the delta. When I wasn't getting snagged, I was pulling up bullheads." I was growing depressed again. A man who finally retires from his daily labors and can go fishing while other people work ought to be able to catch a fish worthy of its name, not ugly green things all head and mouth that I wouldn't want on *my* dinner plate, much less my wife's.

I noticed Millie was sitting across from me quite still, with her hands folded and a peculiar expression on her face. I searched my conscience. Had I forgotten the drop cloth again when I touched up the paint in the living room yesterday? I knew I had cleaned up the boiled-over milk when I fixed my own breakfast early this morning. Millie hates it when I turn the heat up too high under anything on the stove. She says I shouldn't do that and leave the kitchen, because I'm bound not to get back in time to prevent a disaster. She's right, of course. And I have also told her that if she could spend one single day in the middle of the daily flare-ups in my office, she'd never say another thing about my transgressions in the house. That's really not as good an argument as it sounds, though. Millie has worked in an office, too, though not in my line, which was fire insurance.

As I was reflecting on this, she produced some papers that I hadn't noticed were hidden on her lap. Without a word she showed me a page-sized, colored brochure. Oh, it made the tears start in my eyes. There was a picture of a man holding a big salmon by the gills. The caption said: MEL RIEBERS GETS A 34-POUNDER. Below Mel was another picture. In this one, the man was sitting down with a monster fish lying across his thighs. That fisherman wore a grin that probably ruptured his jaw. JERRY LEGGETT WEIGHS IN WITH 70-LB TYEE. A tyee, the brochure explained, was a King salmon weighing up to eighty pounds. The fish looked like a fat, silver-colored submarine with eyes.

Millie waved a smaller brochure. "It's a two-day package off Vancouver Island, British Columbia. Our next-door neighbors, the Vilas, went last year and caught a big one. Arthur, I dare you," she said.

What could I say? Millie had plucked the sadness straight out of my heart, and she knew it. She grinned. "Have some more soup."

The Vilas, as usual, agreed to take in our newspapers and mail, water the plants, and do the things that neighbors do for each

114

other when needed. I said to Burt and Isabel Vila, "If we get an extra fish, can your fridge handle a thirty-pounder?" Both of them laughed and Burt said to Millie, "Oh, have him throw a few back. Leave something for the rest of the fishing party." He sounded patronizing, as usual. Burt thinks he's a wit, and there have been too many times, hours later unfortunately, when I've thought of a wittier comeback.

We flew up to Vancouver, and from the airport transferred to a small plane that took us over some water and then a lot of green forest to Ucluelet, a village on the west side of Vancouver Island. Millie isn't comfortable on planes, especially small ones, but she said not a word in complaint. I held her hand all the way.

What we could see of the village was pretty, but with a two-day package there wasn't time to sightsee. We bedded down early in our room in the lodge by the waterfront. The next morning at six we were on the floating dock waiting to board the ocean-going cruiser, which was firing up its engines. The sun hadn't come up yet. Among other smells I detected the scent of a fishy saltiness. This was the real thing! And there on deck was the crew, every single one a professional who would lead me to the big ones. I squeezed Millie's hand. She was very still, except for her free hand trying to wave off the diesel fumes from the boat's exhaust.

"Are you feeling okay?" Her nod didn't quite convince me. "Once we're aboard we'll be clear of the smoke," I told her, "then you'll have all the fresh air you need."

That's what happened, once we were underway. Along with about ten other fishing customers, Millie and I leaned against the rail and watched the shoreline change shape and widen, then finally disappear.

"The clean, deep ocean," I murmured.

Millie understood what I was referring to. "No rocks to snag on," she said. "No kelp, no rubber tires, no bullheads."

The skipper picked up speed. We were out in the clear and the sun's advance light began to show us where we were, which seemed to be no place. That really excited me. All the better for some real fishing, where the big ones lived.

The skipper cut the engines and we slowed to a stop. The

115

cruiser developed a slight rolling motion, while the wind took hold of the diesel exhaust and blew it over everyone on deck.

Jimmy, our fishing guide, handed out the fishing rods and showed us how to use them. The best thing was the gold and green lure, already attached and ready to go. "No messy anchovies, no squid," I told Millie. She didn't say anything. I took a closer look. Both of her hands gripped the rail; her complexion was like tea leaves after five brewings. She rode each lift and dip of the boat grimly, as if it were a balky elevator. "We shouldn't have come," I said.

"Don't say that!" she snapped. "You have a good time. Get your fish. I want you to catch a nice one to take home." She gave her fishing rod back to Jimmy, patted me on the cheek, and stumbled into the cabin and sat down.

I felt terrible for her. Should I ask the skipper to take us back? I looked at the intent faces of all the other paying customers, jigging their lures up and down in the water, and knew such a request was impossible. I had a feeling that the company expected at least one customer to get unhappy the way Millie was, and to them that was simply too bad. They'd turn back when they were ready. While I was thinking about what to do, someone cried out, "Fish on!"

Jimmy said, "Persons next to him please reel in. Leave him the field."

I watched, excited as the rest. The salmon was a beauty, big and hearty, a bounty of pink meat that I could see through the gills. Its owner, a man about my age, laughed and seemed to want to hold on to it, but of course he had to give it up to Jimmy, who stowed it away in the holding box. "Fifteen pounds," Jimmy said. "Pretty nice."

"Fish on! Fish on!" People were giving the call from all over the boat. I kept on jigging my lure, imagining the flashy brightness of it swooping and diving, imagining it catching the eyes of hundreds of big salmon down there, imagining one extraordinarily big salmon swallowing it.

I had a side view of Millie in the cabin. She hadn't moved; her eyes were shut but I could tell she was far from being asleep.

116

If she was capable of thought at this moment, I was sure it was about solid ground, about lying flat out, even if it was at home on our greasy garage floor, which I had promised months ago to clean up.

There was nothing I could do but continue to jig my lure up and down. Everyone around was getting fish. Well, not everyone, but it seemed that way to me. The man next to me hauled a great big one over the rail. I couldn't understand it. My line couldn't have been more than three feet from his.

At about eleven, Jimmy passed out box lunches. Inside my box was a sandwich, some cookies, and an apple. I went inside to make sure Millie had gotten hers, and she had, though it was obvious to me she had no intention of opening the box. I did it for her, but Millie shook her head and whispered for me to go away, she would be fine.

And so I felt a powerful relief when Jimmy said we were soon going to head for home. All I wanted was for Millie to feel better.

The moment the skipper made a wide turn and opened up, something changed. The rocking motion smoothed out to a fast glide; the freshest air I had ever breathed in my life flew into my lungs. I went into the cabin and coaxed Millie to come out. Within five minutes her entire expression came back to this world, and she was looking around and smiling. She probably also thought I had caught some fish.

When we got back to the dock and Jimmy opened the holding well and showed off the glistening treasure inside to all the people who came to the dock to rubberneck, I had to tell Millie that none of it was remotely mine. Again I felt awful. She deserved to have me catch a fish. She deserved to see a thousand-pound salmon strung up from a hook and me standing beside it. My own disappointment was nothing compared to what she probably felt.

At dinner that night we shared a table with another couple who had been on the boat that day with us. They talked about the three salmon they caught and how, when they got home, they planned to bake, poach, chowder, fry—and for all I knew—fritter some of it and freeze what was left to use for the rest of their lives.

The catching of those fish sounded as though they had personally fought and hauled three Moby Dicks into the boat with their naked hands.

After a silence, perhaps they remembered that we hadn't caught a single fish. Millie opened her handbag and brought out some snapshots. These were of our grandchildren, and even if I believe those kids are sweeter, better-looking, and brighter than anyone else's grandchildren, Millie goes further than that. She can talk anyone under the table about those kids. I knew she was boring the couple—not only boring, but killing the air around us by talking about them. Even the busboy stopped coming to our table to refill our water glasses. Millie has done this to people before; it is a trait of hers that sometimes raises hives on my arms. But tonight I let her go on. I let her have the evening. After what she had gone through for me, I owed her fifty grandchildren to talk about.

In the morning, as I was closing out accounts at the front office, Millie said she had something to do and would be right back. She returned carrying a Styrofoam box. In that box, she said, were two salmon steaks she had bought from the company store for us to take home.

And when we did get home, she didn't fall down and kiss the floor, though I knew she felt like it. That may have been because it was the garage floor. Its layers of grease and dust and leaves sprinkled over the top like cake decorations impressed even me.

What she did do, when she took our diesel-perfumed laundry to the washer downstairs, was give out a squawk that could have been heard in Vancouver. I went to see what had happened.

She was plucking clothes out of the machine; that is, they used to be clothes. Now they looked like the tie-dyed things you saw kids wearing in the '70s. My undershirts had green and red streaks on them, and some other color—I can't find a name for it—that comes when red and green are mixed. Sadly Millie held up a pair of shorts. There seemed to be a picture of a raccoon, done in either red or green, etched into the left leg of the shorts. The right one was an interesting landscape, maybe trees and

118

grass, with a pond in the middle reflecting a violent red sun. The basement smelled as if we were raising mushrooms.

"I'm sorry, Arthur," Millie said. "I did a last load while I was packing for the trip...and I just forgot about it. I'll go right out and buy you new underthings."

"Anyone could have forgotten," I told her, though that calm, even tone of voice took some real effort on my part. "Don't feel bad, honey. That's still good underwear and it wouldn't be the first time, would it?" I've gone around before wearing pink underpants, pink because they had been washed with Millie's red terry cloth bathrobe. According to my wife, sorting colors into separate loads of wash constitutes a waste of good water. I didn't want to know what she had thrown in with my things this time.

That little crisis over, we finished getting settled back into our home. Millie showed me the salmon steaks she had brought back. I was stunned. Our markets never carry any that pink, juicy, or wide around. But those in the market are certainly cheap, considering that these two pieces cost us $500 each.

"Let's give one to the Vilas," she said. "They gave us a piece of their fish when they got back."

After my bragging to Burt, I wasn't anxious to see him. "Maybe they didn't catch one, either. Anyway, what are you going to tell them about that steak?" I asked.

"Don't *worry*," she said. She didn't ask me to go next door with her, and I didn't offer.

I was curious enough, though, to ask her what had transpired at the Vilas' when she returned. "How did it go?"

She emptied, onto the kitchen counter, the grocery bag of newspapers and mail the Vilas had collected for us. "Look, Arthur, here's a letter from Dina. Probably the first chance she's had to write since the kids came down with chicken pox."

Once she started reading mail from our daughter there was no talking to her until she was done. I asked, "Did he laugh, sneer, make a crack?"

"Well, sort of." Millie slit the envelope, unfolded the letter, and started reading.

"What do you mean, sort of?" I asked.

"Oh...um...he said the fish that steak came from must have run to sixty pounds," she replied distractedly. "He said...."

"What? What did he say?" I prodded, not sure I really wanted to know.

She was deep into the letter.

"Millie," I spoke as patiently as I could.

"He said it had to be the biggest bullhead you ever caught, if you caught it at all. So...I told him he should have seen what the others got." She smiled. "I didn't *lie*, Arthur."

I put my arms around my wife and hugged her. Millie and I, we're a team.

Attic Light

by

Lisa Marks Fisher

Empty hat boxes rest here with
head-shaped 60-year-old paper inside
waiting for my grandfather
to return the hat,
but only the hint
of musty cologne mingled with dust
remains. And

I understand why mother keeps them
as she keeps the cedar closets
jammed with Hawaiian honeymoon clothes from '51
and the yellowed wedding dress pressed
against father's suit from his
bluejacket days. Because

at 16, under loose floor boards
I stashed shoe boxes with love letters,

dried corsages and even the cards
ripped to shreds and cried on. We

go to the attic
to peek around passages,
duck-slanted ceilings and walk
through the wedge of luminous dust. Shielding
our faces from cobwebs, we wave
our hands through dancing particles
as if we could re-align the stars

Quest for Nellie

by

Flora A. Scearce

Nana, tell me the story about the lost doll, Billy said.

Nana couldn't stop frying chicken. Instead she turned the pieces over in the skillet, lowered the burner, and put a lid on. As she grabbed a few minutes between that and watching potatoes boiling on a back burner, she pushed a strand of dark hair back with her forearm and rinsed her hands under the spigot.

I've told you that story a hundred times, Billy, she said. And she had. Yet he never tired of listening to it. She always made it new. The doll, Nellie, came vividly to his young imagination and he was spellbound by an era long past when his grandmother suffered hardship as a child in the mountains of North Carolina. She began:

It was the winter of 1920. My father came home to our tiny cabin on the side of Saunook Mountain, walking through icy sludge, his brogans soaked to his feet. When I saw my Poppy, I ran out to meet him, my skinny legs flying. Mommy stood in the doorway holding my little sister, Effie, in her arms. Poppy hugged the three of us, then went over to the open fireplace to warm himself. He pounded his brogans against the fire logs, pulled them off, and sat down with his feet close to the fire.

"Rachel, I need to talk about some things I'm aiming for us to do. Right now I'm hungry as a hound dog," he told my mother.

"Ain't never seed you when you weren't, Jim Wright. I'll git some vittles," she answered.

Mommy had a hard time scurrying up vittles. Our cupboards were nearly bare. There were a few handfuls of cornmeal she'd ground herself, some dried apples, and dried shuckybeans. We had meat on our table only when Poppy caught wild game in his traps.

Poppy's news was that he had found a job at a logging camp. That meant we'd all have to leave right away. We'd have to walk down Saunook Mountain in the snowy cold and could take only what we wore on our backs. Poppy was to meet a Mr. Hoaghan in a place called Celoke. Mr. Hoaghan promised a furnished shanty for us to live in. Later we'd go back and get our belongings.

"Poppy, can I take my doll Nellie?" I begged.

"Honey," he said, "we can't hold onto nothing but each other gitting down the side of this mountain."

Poppy knew how much I loved Nellie. Since we lived miles from the nearest neighbors, she was my only friend. She slept with me and I talked to her like she was real. "We'll come back when this weather lets up," Poppy said.

I cried as we gathered quilts to wrap around ourselves for the trip, tying pieces of flannel around our feet and legs to protect against the snow and cold. I put Nellie's green bonnet on her head and laid her on my tiny cot. Then gently I pulled the covers over her. "I'll come back to get you," I promised.

Nellie was the only doll I'd ever had. Poppy'd dug ginseng root for months before the Christmas that Santa Claus brought her, selling it in town to the manufacturers who used it in medical preparations. It had been our very best Christmas. Mommy made fruitcake from dried apples and pies from pumpkin slices she'd hung above the fireplace to dry. Effie and I had gathered chestnuts and we roasted them in the fireplace.

I'd been thrilled when I found Nellie in my stocking, along with an orange and two peppermint sticks. Afterwards, Mommy took my hand and led me out the cabin door to look at the snow. There were little doll tracks leading up to our door.

"How could Nellie walk in the snow?" I had asked Mommy.

"Santy Claus has magical powers," she'd said. "He held her hand as she walked in the door." Because Mommy told me this, I believed it.

Nellie's head and hands and feet were made of real china. She had painted dark eyes and her ruby lips were in a pouty bow. Brown curls fell below her bonnet. Her green skirt matched the bonnet and there was lace trim on her high-necked blouse.

As Nana told Bill the story, she stopped to check the food.

Why didn't you go back for her, Nana? Bill asked. He knew the answer, but this time he hoped Nana would embellish the story.

Nana took the pieces of chicken from the skillet one at a time, placing them on a layer of paper towels to drain. She went on with her tale:

When we reached the foot of the mountain, we found a blacksmith's shop to rest ourselves and get warm. "We be waiting for a man name of Hoaghan," Poppy told the smith. "He's got a job waiting and a place for us to live."

"That feller's gone away from these parts," the blacksmith said. "The law's after him." The smith told Poppy about another man who was hiring workers for a cotton mill in Greenville, South Carolina.

Poppy found the man and signed up for a job at the mill. He was too proud to tell the cotton mill man we had nothing, but I guess he could see for himself. The man gave Poppy an advance on his wages so we could buy food and clothes and train tickets for Greenville.

Soon my sister and I were going to school. We had new dresses to wear and on Sundays we went to Sunday School. When we were asked to bow for prayer, I remembered that dark night on Saunook Mountain—the snow and ice, and the cabin where my doll, Nellie, lay waiting for me to return. In my prayers I asked God to let some other little girl find Nellie, someone who would care for her as I had.

Do you think some other little girl did find her, Nana? Billy interrupted. He visualized a happy child hugging Nellie.

I hope so, Nana said as she drained the potatoes into the sink and began mashing them. Then she continued the tale.

Mommy never went back to the mountain she loved so well. We had been in the mill village about six months when she died after giving birth to a baby boy. The baby lived only a few days. I was nine years old and Effie was six.

After my father remarried, I asked my stepmother to help me write a letter to my grandmother who still lived near Saunook Mountain. In the letter I asked Granny to find a logger going up Saunook and get him to bring the doll, Nellie, back to her house.

Granny loved Nellie, too. When Effie tore Nellie's collar trying to undress her, Granny fastened it with a brooch Grandpa had given her when they were newlyweds. Nellie wore that brooch from that day on.

Two weeks later, we got an answer to the letter. It was from my Uncle John and written to my father. It stated simply that Granny had died a week before my letter was received. I flung myself on my bed and wept for the dear Granny I loved so much and for my Nellie, the symbol of my lost childhood. I prayed again that someone would find her and love her.

Bill pretended his eye was itching as he brushed away a tear. He always did at this point in her story.

Nana, do you think the doll is still there? he asked.

Oh, no, Honey, she said. *That was over fifty years ago. We never returned to Saunook. I never knew what became of Nellie or our cabin. I doubt the cabin is even still there.* She checked the oven for her biscuits and reset the timer for three more minutes. *Now, go wash your hands and get ready to eat.*

As time passed, Bill thought less about the doll story and his grandmother's roots until college, when he became interested in tracing the family ancestry. That was when he urged Nana to write down all she could remember about her family and her life as it was back then. The project occupied her declining years, until Parkinson's disease took its toll and, no longer able to care for herself, she was moved to a nursing home.

It hurt Bill to see her always bedridden except for brief periods in a wheelchair each day, but he came to see her as often as he could.

"Nana, I'm planning to take you back to Saunook Mountain as soon as I graduate, so I want you to try and get better," he said as he reached for the frail brown-splotched hand.

"I can't go, Bill. I'm just not able." She smiled at the thought of it and he kissed her hand.

"If you don't go with me, I'll have to go alone. I have my journey all mapped out." Bill insisted on showing her the map, though failing eyesight kept her from reading. The planned trip was marked with a heavy yellow line. Tears welled in her eyes and she reached for a tissue stuffed in her sleeve.

She patted his arm. "I love you, Darling."

"I love you, Nana," he said.

Bill's trip was a pilgrimage for Nana. He became her eyes, seeing the green mountain again, with wooden fences zig-zagging through fields of pink and yellow wildflowers kissed by honeybees. He snapped pictures randomly, stopping to chat with farmers. He visited graveyards, copying the names of all the Wrights and Robinsons. He picked wildflowers from Saunook and pressed them between sheets of waxed paper. Drinking in the beauty, he wrote down his impressions to relate to Nana.

She would be here again by proxy. She would know how it felt. She would hear the swift-flowing streams, the thumping of a woodpecker, the dove's lonely cry. She would smell the freshness, feel the breezes, see the shadows as the sun set behind the Smokies. It would all be hers again.

Bill discovered an abandoned cabin in a secluded cove. The door leaned open on rusty hinges. Could this be the one? There was a broken bedstead, a warped table. He thought of Nellie, the doll of Nana's memory. He decided to buy her a doll.

The gift shops in Waynesville abounded with items for the tourist trade. In a quaint shop smelling of mountain potpourri,

Bill browsed through shelves of handcrafted toys, jellies, sour-wood honey, hand-loomed rugs, and found a shelf of dolls.

"I'm looking for an antique doll," Bill explained, and a clerk led him to a back room where dolls reached the ceiling, row on top of row.

His eyes came to rest on an old doll with dark painted eyes on a china face. "That one," he said.

"It's a genuine antique, about eighty years old," the clerk pointed out, as she gently removed the doll from the shelf. "I have other less expensive ones in better condition."

"It doesn't matter," Bill said. "I'll take this one." He pulled out his credit card without asking the price.

Driving up to Guardian Care Nursing Home the following week-end, Bill's heart skipped a beat. He removed his briefcase from the back seat along with the box containing the doll.

A strong odor of pine oil and medication filled the entrance hall where wheelchairs jammed the area near the nurse's station. Given a choice, Nana would be in her room.

As Bill tiptoed in, her eyes were closed. "Nana," he called softly.

She opened her eyes. "Bill?"

"Yes, it's Bill, Nana." She tried hard to smile and held a fee-ble hand out for him to grasp.

"Nana, will you tell me the story about the lost doll?" he asked.

She perked up a little and began shaking her head, pink scalp shining through thinning gray hair. "I've told you that story a hundred times," she said, as if he were a child again.

"Then let me tell it this time," he said.

Bill told of a little mountain girl who had to leave her beauti-ful doll named Nellie, and go down the snowy mountainside from her cabin home, never to return. As he finished the story, a tear slid down her cheek. Pretending her eye was itching, she dabbed it with a tissue.

Tenderly Bill took the doll from the box and held it in front of her.

Her fingers ran over the doll's features and clothes. Then she whispered, "Wherever did you find her?"

"She was still in Saunook, waiting for you to come back for her." Bill's voice trembled as he laid Nellie in the crook of her arm.

Smiling, Nana closed her eyes, crushed the doll to her chest, and went to sleep.

Watching his grandmother's hands begin to shake, Bill looked more closely at the doll. *Could it be?* he wondered.

Sure enough, the doll's green bonnet and skirt were faded at the folds into yellowish gray. Age-darkened lace was ripped slightly above a cameo brooch pinned to her high-necked blouse.

Gone But Not Forgiven

by

Chuck Etheridge

Like most fourteen-year-olds, I was motivated primarily by hormones. So when eighteen-year-old, blue-eyed, red-haired Gail Jones came up to me at church one Sunday and asked me to help her with Vacation Bible School, how could I say no?

After allowing me appropriate time to properly swoon over her glory, Gail gave me more information about our teaching task. Someone, probably the Youth Minister, had gotten the bright idea to combine the Primary (first and second grades) with the Sunbeam (third and fourth grades) class. Gail and I would be charged with the task of teaching twenty rambunctious six-, seven-, eight-, and nine-year-olds.

I began the process of planning Gail's and my wedding, trying to decide which pair of bell-bottoms I would wear to the ceremony. I wasn't listening carefully, but I'm sure she said she wanted me to *help* teach. She also told me that she had a lot of "fun" activities planned—fingerpainting, coloring, singing, and talking about Jesus. "Besides," she said, "we even have a book to follow."

I was wondering what Gail's and my log cabin in the foothills of the Rockies would look like. We would be the envy of all my friends. I would be a nuclear physicist/brain surgeon/pro-foot-ball player. Gail would look on, sighing at all the appropriate moments, and my friends, magically trapped in the tenth grade forever, would gaze on in eternal green envy.

"...so I'll see you on Monday, right?" she asked me.

"Uh, yeah, Gail, sure. I'll be there," I said.

Gail walked away, then turned back. She shot me her dazzling smile, looked at me with those baby blues, and said, "I *really* appreciate this, Chuck." My heart fluttered.

I don't think I gave one thought to the kids in the class or what I was supposed to do. Every thought I had involved me, Gail, and the Beatle Paul McCartney singing "Silly Love Songs" in the background.

Monday came. I entered the classroom and was confronted by a whirling clump of confusion. I later realized that this clump was composed of twenty little kids. I didn't even go into the room; I just stood in the doorway, staring, trying to find Gail in the whirlwind.

Just then, the Vacation Bible School supervisor walked by. "Oh, Chuck, there you are," she said. "Gail just called. She's ill and won't be able to make it today, but she'll be here tomorrow. Let me know if you need any help." Then she vanished.

After a small anxiety attack, I mustered up the courage to enter the room. Eventually the swarm slowed and broke into its individual child parts, which settled down, took seats, and looked up at me, expectantly.

That was when the real panic hit. Alone! I was going to be alone with the kids for hours and hours that day. What would I do? How could I escape with my dignity intact? I had to do a good enough job so that when my goddess, Gail, came to class the next day, she would not banish me from the heaven of her presence.

"H-hi," I stuttered. "I'm Ch-Ch-Chuck. Who are you?" I asked stupidly. A massive explosion of sound erupted as twenty kids screamed their names at the same time.

"Let's try that again. My name is Chuck," I said. "Why don't we go around the room and, one at a time, everybody tell me what your name is."

131

"Hi, I'm Brian. Where's Gail?" came the first response.

"I'm Courtney," said the little girl sitting next to Brian.

Everyone followed in turn. So far, so good, I thought. I'd at least gotten the ball rolling. Then I looked at my watch. Two and a half minutes down, four hours, fifty-seven and a half minutes to go.

Absolute silence descended again as the kids sat and stared, waiting for me to do something teacherly. I stared right back. They started fidgeting. I started fidgeting. I looked at my watch. Four hours, fifty-seven minutes to go.

Inspiration arrived like a bolt from the Deity. "Wanna color?" I asked.

"Yeah!" They even sounded excited.

One of the kids knew where the crayons and papers were kept and passed out the necessary materials. Then the class sat there, Crayolas in hand, staring at me again.

After about three uncomfortable minutes, Brian finally said, "What should we draw?"

Good question. Some part of me still believed that, any minute, Gail was going to walk in the door and whisk me away to a log cabin in a magical land where the second grade didn't exist.

"Why don't you draw...?" I had no idea what they should color. Hey wait! It was Vacation Bible School, right? "Why don't you color *Jesus*?"

They began to color, treating their task like it was assigned by a teacher who had some sense. I even got into the spirit of the thing, grabbed some crayons, and started sketching myself.

After they were done, we all compared our Crayola drawings of Christ. My drawing was, by far, the worst one in the class. Even the first-graders could draw better than I could. Still, the kids were nice to each other and tried to be kind to me, saying things like, "I never thought of giving Jesus green teeth."

I looked at my watch. Four hours, forty-six minutes, thirty-four seconds to go, and we had clearly done all of the drawing we were going to get done. Time to think up a new activity.

"Wanna go outside and play Red Rover?" I asked.

They seemed to think that was a really good idea. We went out on the front lawn of the church and formed two lines of kids.

"Red Rover, Red Rover, let Jenny come over," someone screamed, and a little streak of red and pigtails came hurtling toward our ranks. She broke through, though, and the game started again.

Red Rover kept them busy for, oh, seventeen minutes, thirty-two seconds—although I think their hearts weren't in it during the last three minutes. *Now* what was I going to do?

"It's refreshment time," I bellowed, and we all ran screaming into Fellowship Hall for Hawaiian Punch and Oreos.

When we got there, the punch lady cornered me. "It's not snack time for another hour and a half," she hissed through clenched teeth.

"I am fourteen years old and I have just been thrown at the mercy of twenty small children, and I have no idea what I'm doing. I want some cookies *now!*" I demanded. I got the cookies and, since I had stood up against the evil punch lady, was a hero to the kids.

We had contests to see who could think up the most original way to eat an Oreo, drank punch until our bellies were ready to explode, and staggered back up to the classroom so I could inflict some more boredom on them.

"Wanna read the *Bible?*" I tried to say "Bible" so it sounded really appealing.

"Noooooooooooooooo," came the overwhelming consensus.

I tried to read the Bible to them anyway. Mistake. The more I read, the more like zombies they got. Being the keen lad that I was, it finally dawned on me that the King James Version was not going to appeal to six-year-olds. Time to think of another activity.

The whole day went like that. We'd fingerpaint something vaguely theological, then we'd go climb on the monkey bars. Inside we'd head to get some more snacks and consume them guiltily under the evil glare of the punch lady. Then back to the room to cut out construction paper Noah's Arks, before another round of Red Rover.

Early the next day, the Vanishing Vacation Bible School Supervisor materialized before my door, gave me her plastic smile, and said, "Gail is sick and won't be able to be here. But she said she'll be sure to be here tomorrow." Then she dematerialized.

The whole week went pretty much like the first day. I would desperately scramble for things the kids could do, take them outside a lot, take a ton of snack breaks, vanquish the evil punch lady, and then do some more of the same. If nothing else, I kept my students entertained. No parents complained, or if they did, I never heard about it. The kids seemed to have a pretty good time. Even I survived, and I don't think I did the kids any permanent damage.

On about the fourth day I began to wonder whether or not Gail had ever intended to show up at all. I wondered if it all hadn't been part of a plot hatched by her, Mrs. Vanishing Supervisor, and the evil punch lady, who together had conspired to throw me at the mercy of the throng of cookie-hungry elementary school kids.

I didn't worry about it for long, though. Class would interrupt my daydreaming and I'd have to wipe a nose or break up the fight over who got to use the umber and yellow-orange crayons.

Still, Gail had flashed me that spectacular smile and looked at me with those deep blue eyes, and part of me kept hoping she would show up. Now, after a decade and a half and the demise of bell-bottomed pants, I've decided that our wedding is definitely off. But maybe justice was served. Gail eventually turned into an evil punch lady herself who has to deal with jerks like me during Vacation Bible School.

Life and Love and Chocolate Sodas

by

Betty Gray

If you happen to be near Bastrop, Texas on a Wednesday afternoon about two o'clock, drive down Main Street, park as near as
you can to Lock's Drugs and come on in! Most likely you'll see
me there sitting at one of those little round wooden tables, contentedly sipping my soda through a straw.

No, this is no ordinary soda. This is the kind of soda a real
chocolate lover dreams of. This is a *thick* chocolate soda with chocolate ice cream stirred into it so that you have to almost *pull* the
potion through the straw. And, of course, it's topped with a huge
glob of whipped cream with a big red cherry carefully balanced
on the top just right. But be careful; you have to lift the cherry off
ever so gracefully with the long-handled spoon or the cherry will
hop right off the whipped cream onto the table or, even worse,
clear down to the floor to be lost forever.

Now, this soda mania of mine did not originate with me.
Oh, no. It has been passed down to me through my genes. Way
back there in time, a mutant gene of the "Chocolate Soda Type I"
strain appeared in our family's otherwise normal genetic pattern.
I have now traced the active "C.S." gene back as far as my grand-

135

father's generation. And it only appears on my mother's side of the family.

Looking back on my annual childhood visits to Arkansas with my grandparents, I realize that Papa's generation was deeply affected by the action of this strange mutation. Let me explain further.

On those lazy summer mornings as my brother, my cousins and I lay sleeping on our quilt-beds on the living room floor, we were awakened—gradually and unwillingly—by Nana's and Papa's "try-not-to-wake-the-children" whispers. They were making plans for our day.

Now, my grandfather was not only a Methodist preacher, but he was also a clever man. He wanted his grandchildren to know that life would not always be easy, and that hard work could reap many fulfilling rewards. Each day we were offered "opportunities" through which we could earn money to purchase an item of our choice at their small town's hub of activity and news, the Main Street Soda Fountain and Pharmacy.

Papa's favorite summer money-earning challenge for us was fly-swatting. Now, if you've ever been in Arkansas in the summer, you know that there are *plenty* of flies thriving in all that heat and humidity. We'd just sit on the big porch swing or on the porch steps and swat our prey with great vigor. We would swing and swat and then swing and swat, but those Arkansas flies were *fast* and those flies were *smart.* For each batch of five flies, we were paid three cents. Most days, from a whole morning's swatting, we'd earn enough to buy a one-dip cone. Sometimes we'd save up a few days earnings and put it together with a cousin's and then buy a great big soda with a straw for each contributor. Nothing in the world was more worth our investment than those sodas!

As we grew older and wiser, we realized that we had learned a valuable lesson about work and sharing and love. It was great to have a grandfather who was affected by the wonderful Chocolate Soda Syndrome.

When I was a little older and wiser and more understanding, my mother confided that her plans for her life had also been altered by the C.S. Syndrome. Her symptoms, she said, began surfacing in 1919, the year she graduated from college.

Mother had every intention of being a music teacher in the Fordyce, Arkansas public schools. She had even signed a contract for three years—a rash step for a young lady in those days. To celebrate her entry into the world of business, she strolled downtown, entered the Main Street Soda Fountain and Pharmacy—and that was when fate intervened. On the stool next to her sat a handsome young man in uniform. He had just graduated with the first class of pilots from the newly formed United States Army Flight School at Chanute Field. The Armistice had just been signed and he had just ordered a chocolate soda to celebrate his release from military service.

He took one look in my mother's direction and he ordered another soda. This one was for her. He didn't even know her name; she was just a perky little redhead seated beside him.

Of course he then properly introduced himself to her. He told her about his plans to enter the insurance business, probably down in Little Rock. Over the next month or so, more sodas were shared. Before long, the reliable old Chocolate Soda Syndrome caused my mother to go to the Fordyce Superintendent of Schools with a request to withdraw from her contract.

The Superintendent was very patient and understanding—perhaps he'd had a few chocolate sodas himself. The redhead and the young insurance man married and that's where I entered into the picture—three years later.

Now let's skip down through the years; the clock has ticked around to the 1940s. We are now in Houston, Texas and these are the years of World War II. And the genetic oddity persists.

I was a student at Rice University. My family lived near the school, so there was never an option for me to go to school anywhere else. Through his will, William Marsh Rice had made it possible for students to attend the university tuition-free. What a fine situation! My family did not come out financially ahead, however. But it wasn't my fault; it was that C.S. Syndrome at work again. It caused me to spend more time at the soda fountain over at the Episcopal Church's student center on Main Street than I did in class. And I probably spent more money on chocolate sodas and such than I would have for tuition! After all, there were 100 girls at Rice and 600 boys. How could a girl study?

Now, into the picture came a new element. Right down the street from my family's home was a house that belonged to a nice widow with four children. She also provided bed and breakfast for two "reliable young working men." One of these young men was an aspiring architectural engineer from "deep East" Texas. He was working in Houston while waiting to be notified if his name came up on the list of candidates for pilot training in the United States Air Force. Yes, this was the World War II era.

Well, the teenage sons in the widow's house told the girl student about the about-to-be-pilot and vice versa. There was some curiosity, but not too much hope. After all, the pilot-to-be didn't have time to waste on a silly young girl. And the young girl had all the dates she was allowed to have.

Eventually they met. The young man was very tall. His legs were very long and his shoes were very large. The words bounced out of her mouth all by themselves, "You surely do have big feet!" She wanted to die. So did he.

"I'm sorry," she said. "It's just that my dad's feet are very small."

"Would you like to go for a soda?" he asked, gratefully changing the subject.

Now how could he possibly know sodas were her favorite thing in the whole world? "I guess so," she replied. She waved goodbye to her startled mother as the two of them—strangers to each other—walked toward the soda fountain a few blocks away. And there it was, that C.S. Syndrome hard at work again.

Eventually this very different young man received his long-awaited orders to report to the Santa Ana Air Force Base. His training continued at several other bases. To the college girl, waiting anxiously at home, this time seemed like it lasted forever.

The young man illustrated his letters to her with clever little cartoons depicting every phase of his life as a "hot pilot." The college girl found herself more and more fascinated by this man whom she had come to know intimately through their correspondence.

138

After it seemed like it would never happen, he came home on leave. Now this is the point when the Chocolate Soda Syndrome performed another great miracle.

The young couple drove into downtown Houston to attend a special movie. In those days, before television, movies were *the* visual entertainment. There were two theaters side by side on Main Street. Certainly the couple would be able to get into one of them. But, no. They had to purchase their tickets and then wait for the next feature. Happily there was a great candy store next door with a soda fountain.

They found an empty booth and ordered *one* chocolate soda with *two* straws. The young woman had matured quite a lot while this man was away. She now knew that more was not necessarily better. Why, she would rather be with this one man than all of those 600 boys at Rice. So, there they sat, gazing into each other's eyes.

The crowd was beginning to come out of the theater. The couple swallowed their last sips of soda and went over to join the line of people waiting to hand their tickets to the usher so they could get into the movie theater right away.

As they reached the front of the line the young man reached into his pocket to retrieve the ticket stubs. Oh, no! In his nervousness and excitement of being with the girl he had waited so long to find, he had shredded the theater tickets into bits! The young man shrugged his shoulders, the usher smiled, and the couple turned away, laughing, to walk back out into the night. The movie wasn't really that important any more.

Here we are now, almost 50 years later. The Chocolate Soda Syndrome still persists relentlessly. The moment our children, and especially our grandchildren, walk in the door on their visits with us, they blurt out, "Is the soda fountain open today?" So, off we go, down to the little Main Street of our retirement town, to Lock's Drugs for a soda. Now how's that for having it all?

And may the Chocolate Soda Syndrome flourish forever!

Jack

by

Barbara Lucey

Your grandfather took very good care of himself, you can say that
for him. Now I'm not saying he was a selfish man, but Jack always
came first with Jack. He made sure he ate right, starting with a
breakfast of oatmeal, a boiled egg, bread and butter, stewed
prunes, and his tea. Then Marie packed his lunch, two ham sandwiches—"sang-wiches" he called them—ham sliced so thin by
Charlie at the market on Martin Street that he'd cut his fingers
when he sliced it. Just so Jack could have two slices per sandwich,
make him feel like a rich man. A piece of fruit, some A&P raisin
cookies, the kind that were pressed completely flat—you remember them, whatever they were called, Golden Fruit, was that it? I
can't remember names anymore.

   And I'm sure he had a shot at lunchtime, too. I know because I was there, that's how. In the summertime, sometimes
Marie would send me down to the hospital boiler room with a
slice of angel food cake she'd just made, or a bottle of homemade
root beer or a note—they were still in love then—and I'd stick
around while he and Bert what's-his-name would play checkers.
They had a bottle, sure, but Jack—that was his gift—he could always take just one and jeez, how he'd enjoy it. Stand up with the
glass in his hand, give a toast to the furnace, shouting something

over it like, "To hell with you, you bastards." It was really a roar in there, that's how he went deaf. Well, you know that. Then he'd throw it all down in one swig and smile with his teeth, like this, letting out a big blast through them, saying, "Hah!" He'd smash the glass down on the checkerboard and all the pieces would jump. Now, why would he need more than one of those, I ask you.

And of course, he walked everywhere. That's why he stayed fit to the end. We had a car for a while in the thirties, a Dodge. But he'd hardly ever drive it and eventually he sold it. We'd take Uncle Pat's car for trips to visit the Manchester clan or to the beach, once in a while for a ball game in Pittsfield. Jack wasn't an especially good driver and Jack didn't enjoy doing anything he wasn't good at, so hang the rest of us if we thought we needed a car. There was the expense of course, too, but that wouldn't have mattered to Jack if he had thought a car was necessary, necessary to the old man, that is.

It was the middle of the Depression—cardboard soles in our shoes—but we had meat for dinner every night—chops, a roast, a little daisy ham—and chicken every Sunday, or a pot roast. That to Jack was what living in America was all about. Without meat on his family's table and in his belly, he wouldn't be a man. He might as well go back to Ireland and have his tea and toast with a wee bit of milk, and meat once a month.

Most evenings—but not all the time—he'd have a bottle of beer which I'd bring up from the cellar for him or Joe would, or Edmund, sometimes with a shot. And he'd read his paper at the kitchen table, wetting his index finger and thumb to turn the pages, telling us all the news of the world. Very well informed, Jack was, right up into his nineties, reading two papers a day and his *Reader's Digest* every month. Didn't want to be caught off guard. The news of the world and mathematics, he prided himself on those. Remember how he used to always test you kids with math problems—do 'em in your head. Twenty-five times three hundred and forty. Ah, but Jack had to be the smartest one, always had to let you know he was the clever one. He was actually disappointed if you got it right so he couldn't crow "Aha!" over your head and thump on his chest.

141

From Kerry, he could have gone on to school in Dublin, you know. They'd offered him a scholarship. Not Jack, though. Ireland was finished for him. He wanted a place of his own, some nice clean painted boards and a truck garden, a town, a little technology. A future, you see. It was all dead for him there—the priests, the old maids and bachelors.

Well he got his life and a good long one, too. I guess probably just about the way he'd pictured it.

Tumbleweed Christmas

by

Robert and Jean Flynn

Lucille stepped from the long, yellow school bus and walked
slowly down the dirt road toward home. She pulled her too-short
coat closer around her, but she couldn't protect her thin, uncovered legs from the cold, biting, sand-filled wind that blew against
them. It was the last day of school before Christmas.

She looked at the flat, brown land, empty of life for the winter and felt the same emptiness inside herself. Her father didn't
want Christmas in the house. "You're too big for a tree," he said.
He didn't want any of it—not the carols, or the wreaths, or even
the joy. Not since Lucille's mother had died.

Although she was only twelve, Lucille understood that it was
not because her mother had died, but because her father hadn't
been able to give her anything while she was alive. The house
wasn't their own. They had no car. Their clothes were worn and
second-hand. But Lucille knew that her mother had been happy.
Her mother had had the liveliest eyes in town. Everyone said that.
Eyes that sparkled like lights on a Christmas tree. Thinking about
her mother's eyes made Lucille want to cry.

Lucille put her books and the gift-wrapped package she had
brought from school on the table. She didn't have time to cry.
She had to clean the house, tend the animals, and fix supper.

143

Like her mother, Lucille didn't mind hard work. "Hands that can't find work can't find ease either," her mother used to say.

For a long time after he hurt his back working on Mr. Walser's barn, her father could not get a job. He went from house to house all day asking for any kind of work. Lucille took care of the cow and the chickens and the pigs, the house and the garden, and her mother cleaned and ironed for other people.

"I'm going to make it up to you," he kept saying to them both. "You'll see. Christmas is going to come." It seemed like he had been saying that for as long as she could remember. But it wasn't his fault. When he got a job at the meat-packing house there was a difference in the way he came home, in the way he said, "Christmas is going to come this year."

Then her mother got sick, and in spite of all the doctor could do, she died. It started all over again—her father with no light in his eyes, not even a promise of Christmas this year.

"You're too big for birthdays," he said. Why couldn't he realize that she would never be too big for Christmas trees and birthdays, but that she was big enough to understand why he couldn't give her a present? Why couldn't he just say, "Happy Birthday" or "Merry Christmas" and smile at her again.

Just as she couldn't stop the west Texas wind from blowing, she couldn't stop the tears from falling. She hung her cup towel over the sink to dry and grabbed the bucket to go milk. She angrily brushed the tears aside.

The tears went away but the anger did not, and when Old Brown kicked at the milk bucket, Lucille hit the cow in the flank. When the chickens got so excited they turned over their pan and spilled all the feed, she lashed out at them, too.

"Why does he have to be so mean to himself?" she asked the pigs. "There'll be no Thanksgiving in this house," she mimicked her father. She had known there wouldn't be turkey. She didn't even like turkey. She knew he wouldn't kill a hen; he'd sold all the culls. She just wanted them to eat together, but he had volunteered to work that day because they needed the money. He had come in too tired to eat. Lucille had eaten alone. She was glad when Thanksgiving was over and she could go back to school.

Lucille liked school. She liked reading about other places and learning new things. Reading poetry was her favorite because it made her insides sparkle like Mama's eyes had. But the first time she had looked into a microscope was almost as exciting. And so was learning about Thomas Jefferson and Joan of Arc. She wished she could stay in school forever, even if some of the children made fun of her clothes.

"You should never be embarrassed about your clothes as long as they are mended, clean, and ironed," Mama used to say. Lucille hadn't been, except for the time Papa had seen her in one of Mama's dresses. She wasn't embarrassed exactly, but it felt like being embarrassed.

It was a special day in the school, the day for school pictures, and she had wanted a special dress. She had opened her mother's closet and there Mama's things were, as though she were still alive. She had chosen the blue polka dot dress with the velvet ribbon which she could adjust by rolling up the sleeves and tying the ribbon tightly around her waist. She had thought Papa wouldn't mind, and he hadn't exactly. He mistook her for her mother. "Rosa," he had said, and his voice conveyed his shock of happiness, but his face betrayed the disappointment that it was Lucille in Rosa's dress.

"I'm sorry, Papa," she said, but he couldn't look at her, not when she was wearing her mother's dress, and he seemed unable to speak to her about her mother. Later he would not allow her to help as he packed her mother's things to take to the church for the needy. "There are those who need them more than you," he said and she nodded. She knew that he did not want to be reminded of Mama every time he saw her dresses. But she wished he would talk to her about Mama.

Lucille set the heavy bucket of milk on the table and looked at the package that was already covered with a fine coat of dust. What was she going to do with her Christmas present for Papa? All the children made Christmas presents for their parents at school. She wished she had explained to her teacher why she couldn't give Papa a gift. She was afraid of being embarrassed in front of her class by telling the teacher her father couldn't afford a present for her and her gift to him would make him unhappy.

Besides, it wasn't just a present for Papa, it was a present to her from the teacher. The teacher gave the children a school picture of themselves and the end of an orange crate to decorate as the picture frame. She brought scraps of paper, cloth, and paint to the school. Lucille had made a background out of the soft, cushiony paper from a candy box.

Some of the boys heated metal rods and burned designs into the rough wooden crate frame. Some of the girls brought satin or flannel from home and glued it to the frame. Lucille decided to paint hers. There were only two kinds of paint—cowbarn red and locomotive black. The Murphy twins wanted the red and Lucille knew better than to argue with them. She painted hers black. Out of old magazines, she cut out pictures of the things she loved—horses, dogs, elephants, rabbits, and bluebonnets. The other children laughed, but her teacher said it was original and gave her a gold star to glue to the top of the frame.

Lucille liked the picture of herself in Mama's dress, surrounded by the things she loved, with a bright gold star over her head. But she remembered the look on Papa's face and hid the package under clothes in a drawer. She would decide later what to do with it.

On Christmas Eve, Lucille went about her chores singing carols all day. Maybe Papa would walk to town with her like they used to with Mama to see the lights and decorations, and hear the music, and look in the windows, and watch the children in their excitement and expectations.

Papa was finishing the meal Lucille had prepared before going to milk when she returned to the house. "Lucille, I'm going to have to go back to work tonight and will work a shift tomorrow. It means you will be home alone on Christmas Day, but we need the money."

Lucille busied herself putting away the milk so Papa wouldn't know how disappointed she was. "Yes, Papa," she said.

"I'm going to go now," he said.

"Can I go too, Papa?" she asked without thinking.

146

"No," Papa said. "I'm going straight to work. I won't be coming home."

"Please, Papa," she said. "I can walk home by myself." This plea just came out of her mouth. He thought she would be disappointed seeing all the things she couldn't have, but she wouldn't be. She just wanted to be a part of Christmas for a little while.

"I don't have time," he said.

She didn't cry until after he was gone.

There were no tears Christmas Day when Lucille began her chores. She was a big girl, almost a woman, and what did Christmas mean but thinking of others beside herself.

She knew what she would do. She would have a Christmas party for the animals and give herself the picture she had made at school. She would fix little presents for Old Brown, and for the hens, and the chickens, and the pigs. She would invite them all to the barn, sing carols to them, and give them their presents.

She wished she had a Christmas tree. Any kind of tree would do. Even the limb off a tree would do. But they had no trees except the pecan tree and she dared not break a limb off the pecan tree. Papa picked up the pecans and sold them, but he would never thrash the limbs or allow her to climb into the tree and shake its branches.

"The pecan tree is good to us," Papa said. "What kind of people would we be if we hurt it by taking its presents?"

She had given up on the tree when she noticed the tumbleweeds that had blown up against the garden fence.

A tumbleweed Christmas tree.

All morning Lucille worked building and decorating the tumbleweed Christmas tree. She almost burst with excitement choosing just the right tumbleweeds and carrying them one by one to the barn where she had cleared a place for her party. She put three tumbleweeds together for the base, then two and then one small one for the top, until it was the biggest tree she had ever seen.

She cut the star off the chicken feed sack and stuck it on top. Old Brown's rope was not the color she preferred, but she wrapped it around the tree several times. She found some plastic rings that Papa had used when he culled the hens and hung them on the stems of the tumbleweeds. Then she shelled some corn and cut the corn cobs in round slices and hung them for balls.

Lucille ran to the house, for once not minding the cold wind that chapped her face and stung her legs. She had forgotten all discomforts in her excitement about her Christmas party. She took a box from the closet shelf where Mama had saved used wrapping paper and bows and carefully chose three pieces of paper with bows to match.

Back in the barn she wrapped her little presents of shelled corn for the pigs, bread crumbs for the chickens, and a cotton-seed cake for Old Brown.

Lucille placed the presents for the animals along with her own under the tumbleweed Christmas tree, then brought the animals to the barn and sang carols to them. Old Brown listened while patiently chewing her cud, the chickens eyed the presents with curiosity, but Lucille had to scold the pigs because they were interested in nothing but what was under the tree.

Lucille was having so much fun she didn't know when Papa entered the barn. She might not have noticed him at all except that Old Brown stopped chewing and the chickens turned their curiosity from the presents to the barn door. The pigs did not seem to notice Papa at all, and when Lucille saw him and stopped singing, they rushed in, tore the packages, and ate some of Old Brown's cottonseed cake before Lucille was able to chase them away. "Mean old pigs," she said, close to tears.

Papa sat down beside her and put his arms around her. The pigs kept their distance, looking over their shoulders. They were afraid of Papa.

"I was going to give the animals their presents and the pigs ruined it all," she said.

Papa tidied up the packages, smoothing out the torn paper and rewrapping the cottonseed cake.

"There," he said, "whose present is this?"

"Old Brown's," Lucille said.

Papa opened the torn package and gave the cake to Old Brown. "And whose present is this?"

148

"The pigs'," Lucille said.

"Let's make them wait until last," Papa said, taking the other package and spreading the bread crumbs for the chickens. Only then did he notice that there was an extra present and looked at Lucille. She couldn't speak. "I'll bet this is for me," he said. He gave the corn to the noisy pigs before opening his gift.

"It's a beautiful frame, and a beautiful picture of a beautiful girl and I'm going to keep them forever," he said. He hugged her and kissed the top of her head.

Then he reached into his pocket and pulled out a little package wrapped in silver with red ribbon and a red bow. "Whose present is this?" he asked. It was the prettiest thing Lucille had ever seen, but she could not speak. "It must be for you," Papa said, placing it in her hand.

"Oh, Papa, thank you, it is so pretty," she said, thinking how much such paper and ribbon must cost. She held it to her cheek.

"Aren't you going to open it?" Papa asked.

Lucille couldn't believe it. There was another present inside. "I don't want to tear it," she said, a tear trickling down her face. The package was too perfect to spoil.

Papa slipped the bow from the package and put it in her hair. He took off the ribbon and tied it around her wrist. He unwrapped the paper and smoothed it and placed it on the ground beside her. He handed her a blue velvet box that was the prettiest thing she had ever seen.

She took the box in her hand, feeling the soft fur of the velvet, and held it to her cheek. "Open it," Papa said. Lucille couldn't believe it. Inside the box was yet another present. Slowly she opened the box, and inside the box on a bed of satin lay a beautiful gold watch with a leather band.

It was the most beautiful watch she had ever seen, so beautiful it frightened her. It was not a watch like any of the other children had. It was not a watch for a little girl. Lucille was confused. She could only stare at it. Papa took the watch and placed it on her wrist. Then he hugged her tight.

"I was going to give it to your mother," he said. "I put it on layaway last Christmas because I wanted her to have something

149

fine. I worked overtime to pay for it so I wouldn't take anything away from you. When she was sick, I asked the jeweler to let me take it for a little while so she could see it, so she would know that this year Christmas was going to come. She said that you and me, we were the only Christmas she ever needed."

Papa stopped and Lucille thought he was going to cry. Instead he scolded the pigs that were trying to get the last of the chickens' bread crumbs.

"Oh, Papa," Lucille said, giving him a kiss. She looked just in time to see one of the pigs take the beautiful silver wrapping paper in its mouth. One of the other pigs tried to take it away, tearing it. But Lucille did not cry. She remembered what it was like when it was perfect.

Home

by

Cheryl Kerr

It is always fall in my memories of going home. The crisp, clear weather, red leaves, and wood smoke are part of returning to the fold, of family.

This fall I will take my daughter home for the first time. She is the fourth generation, born in March, the continuity of our blood.

Home is my grandmother's, Hanna's great grandma, a stone house on a graveled drive under century-old poplars and pecans, fronting a comfortably leaning garage. Here we, my mother, aunts, cousins, and I gather in remembrance of our shared history and love for each other.

Perhaps home is a ritual because it is not often done. My mother, aunt, and I, and now Hanna, leave in the gray light of dusk on the journey; the drive is long, flat, and well-worn at this stage of my life. As a child I memorized the towns to break its monotony. This trip seems to have arrived so quickly; I packed for two days and left still not feeling ready. A new mother.

The litany of towns unfolds ahead of us as night falls. Winking lights spread across the dark miles, shadowing horses and cattle in the passing fields. We drive on, greenly lit by the dash lights, talking softly. Hanna sleeps with the intentness of babyhood, her fists curled with the effort.

Our turn looms suddenly from the dark, the first road past the cemetery, stony and rough. Spitting, popping gravel announces our arrival. The porch light shines and below it is Gran's face, anxious and waiting. She hurries to meet us, saying, "I thought you were never coming. I just knew you'd changed your minds," trying to see us all at once.

Quiet descends as I lift Hanna from her seat. Roused from sleep by voices, she looks foggily around and then grins delightedly at my grandmother. I hand her over and they smile at one another, Hanna reaching to touch her cheek. A heart-tugging moment filled with love, expectancy, and wisdom all present.

A flurry of hugs and greetings follow as we troop inside. Hanna is argued over. Who will carry her? Feed her? Where will she sleep? Laughter replies to the query of who will change her. We settle around the table as coffee is brought, strong and dark. The night closes in around us, sighing through the trees overhead as we talk late, catching up, reminiscing, dreaming.

Polished wood and Desert Rose dishes catch pieces of light creating a myriad of tiny reflections of each of us, diffused and soft. Hanna has long since gone to bed, her playpen set as a compromise in the middle bedroom, which, in this old house, opens into all the other rooms. A dog barks and we realize the lateness of the hour, especially for my grandmother who rises with the sun. Quilts and pillows are piled and ready for us. I choose to sleep by the fire and watch the flames. When Hanna wakes I will feed her by its light, soft and warm and lulling.

I step outside to check the car and glimpse the cemetery resting quietly in the moonlight. Sight of it sends the familiar chill down my back. As a child I was terrorized by my cousins and their ghost stories, real and imagined. A favorite trick was the ironing board set in the wall of the back room, my room when I came. The door would creak slowly open and the board come crashing down, draped in an old dress or sheet, sending me into tears, screaming for someone to come. It is a peril to be the youngest grandchild.

The stars are bright here, reminding me of ice chips in the chill night air. I return to the house, glad of the others. Perhaps I will sleep next to the fire for comfort.

As I flick off the last lamp, porch light filters dimly into the room. This light burns always, a custom from my grandmother's youth when it welcomed lonely and weary travelers. To me, it still does.

Nights are cold on the edge of the hill country and the pungent, spicy smell of cedar steals in. Sleep comes easily as I snuggle into the quilts.

Bed springs creak it seems moments later; five o'clock, rising time. I awaken next to the murmur of voices and smell of coffee. From the kitchen doorway a gleam of light reveals Gran, Mom, and my aunts remembering their own childhood and youth.

Shivering, I crawl from bed to check on Hanna, and am met with bright eyes and a toothless smile. She, in her short life, has never slept much past daybreak, surely not if others are up.

We bundle up and she and I greet the dawn from the front porch. As I savor sunrise through the trees and still falling dew, she pats her quilt and coos at the leaves. Sunrise, to me, is anticipation of things to come, a day yet untracked. I wonder what this day will bring. It is really Hanna's. Her chance to be marveled at and known. Beyond the road, haze rises from the river bottom to meet the sun. The others join us and we share the steps and sunrise. All are quiet. Some moments do not need words.

Beckoned by the smell of bacon escaping the house, we go in to breakfast. There are platters of food; Gran thinks we come to eat; this morning we do not disappoint her.

The day is beautiful, cool and breezy, lit by clear bright sunshine. Hanna rolls and tumbles across the yard as though she made the day. Skittering autumn leaves send her into a tailspin of excitement as she chases them, she and a fuzzy kitten, batting at each other among the drifts.

My baby pictures are strewn about, the center of a long discussion of Hanna and me. Our resemblance is strong, the eyes and the smile most of all. And a look of having the world by the tail. Saucy, my grandmother says. I have learned some things the hard way for it, as will she, my child.

My grandmother sits beneath a tree in a semicircle of garden chairs set out for company. She has sat thus since my earliest memories of home began. I remember coming up the road at a gallop and sliding to a stop in front of her, just, my horse blowing, seeing her calm-eyed smile. She was raised with horses and raised mine from a foal, sweet but ready to run. I still miss my mare with the unreasonable anger that death evokes in children. I was not ready to say goodbye. Gran knows this. From across the others, she catches my eye and smiles. They say we are alike.

At sunset we watch the hills deepen into purple and black. Softly and then night, suddenly, is here. Our twilights are hazy and purple-smudged, made so by the cedar. Our violet crown it is called. The day has had that curious, crystal quality that will make it a halcyon memory, magical and bright, with no discordant notes.

A quick hug and steady-eyed smile from my favorite aunt, usually so undemonstrative, brings me from my reverie. She feels it, too. Dawn and twilight bring peace and reflection here. As the daylight dwindles it draws us together, confidences and closeness coming easier.

Hanna is quiet as I ready her for bed, only her eyes move as she lies in my lap. A day of play and strange surroundings has worn her out.

Supper conversation centers around the family members who came by today. And those new to the family cemetery; so many have gone this year. There is a timeless feel as we talk. Tonight we are old and comfortable together, past last night's excitement of arrival.

Always before I have come home as the granddaughter, the youngest, and have listened to the others telling and retelling our past, weaving our family tapestry. Tonight, though, I am aware of an indefinable shift in roles. No longer just a listener, I am now a storyteller, and am fulfilling my own role, continuing our family and traditions in my daughter, Hanna.

There is gentle laughter as I tell them of Hanna's first real giggle, on Mother's Day of this year. My first.

These faces are so much a part of what I value. Their strength is deep and enduring, intertwining us with gnarled but velvet ties. The years have held their challenges for each of us and I meet mine with the gift of this place and these people. This gathering, and yester ones, is a pilgrimage to our past, our present, and most of all, to ourselves.

Tomorrow we will return to our different lives, perhaps questioning their separateness. But tonight, this weekend, is to be shared and cherished, a tribute to our ancestry and heritage.

I make many trips home in my mind. It is a spiritual journey to a time and place that rests my soul.

"Down a gravel road lies a small stone house. And in the doorway a woman waits, sunlight glinting from her hair and glasses. Overhead a poplar drops its first leaves as fall approaches, cool and bright."

That picture rests always in my mind and heart—home. Forever on the edge of time and memory.

A Tangled Web

by

Phoebe Newman

My writing career really began the summer that Grandaddy ran off to Eufaula and had his sex change. He came home in an awful print dress and white wedgies, smelling like gardenia powder and wearing an Eva Gabor wig that had definitely spent some years in a Goodwill Store.

This was the same Grandaddy who used to mow the grass in his pajama bottoms and shame us all to death. He had become a little peculiar since Grandma ran off, but this was just the limit! What would we say at school if they asked us about our family? What if we had to draw a family tree?

Nina and Bubba and I stayed under the porch or up in the trees a lot that summer, trying to avoid the whole thing.

We avoided it, but Momma acted like it never happened. Her own daddy! She absolutely refused to call him anything but Irene, and insisted we did, too. *Miss* Irene. She told people that her own sweet daddy passed away while on a coon shoot up in Dahlonega, and had been buried in the fields of his family homestead. An outright lie! But Momma went right ahead and bought a Stone Mountain granite tombstone and had it shipped off to north Georgia.

The fact that we hadn't even been notified in time to go to

the funeral just proved Momma's lifelong claim that all of our north Georgia relatives were tacky and spiteful.

Irene was supposed to be Grandaddy's maiden sister, who, for all these years, had lived up North, and now had finally come home to stay just when her only blood relative took it into his head to die out in the middle of some piney woods.

Naturally Momma took her in, made her feel right at home and would not listen to one word of argument about where she would sleep and eat for the rest of her days. She was going to eat at our kitchen table with us and sleep in what used to be Grandma and Grandaddy's room. Needless to say, she fit right in. She even took to wearing some of Grandma's things she found in the back of the chifforobe. They did not hang gracefully on her.

Momma told us a hundred times, "This is family business. If I ever hear that one of you children has said a word to anybody in this town, I will switch you 'til you dance!"

Lordy, it was a hard time! Especially as it became obvious that the "change" that Grandaddy went through in Eufaula had been more of a spiritual conversion than an actual medical procedure. We tried to look unconcerned as Irene's beard grew back in beneath her pancake makeup.

It was extra hard, too, because Momma had always fussed at us for telling lies—even the teensiest white lies. The way she kept tabs on our honesty was by reading our diaries, listening in on our phone calls, and walking into our rooms any time she felt like it.

I had a real trying summer recording the strange goings-on in our house, and hiding my diary from Momma. Finally I started keeping two sets; one about boys and dresses and spend-the-night parties for her to read, and one about the truth, which I kept hid in a ditch.

We kids felt sure that when Daddy came home from being out on the road, he would straighten the whole thing out in five minutes flat. But when he did come home one evening, right after we had cut into a watermelon out on the back porch, he just took the heart of the fruit, sat down on the glider and said, "Well, Miss Irene, how's it going?" Serious as all get out. We stood there with our mouths hung open, stunned.

As the days hummed by, Nina and Bubba and I watched with fascination as Irene made her way into the community. The Garden Club, the Circle, the Auxiliary all welcomed her; such was the persuasion of my momma's unquestioned reputation for honesty among the ladies of our town.

Grandaddy's old buddies from the bowling team and the church choir just looked everywhere but at us when we met them on the street. They looked shame-faced and confused. I reckon we did, too.

The July day the mailman brought the letter for Grandaddy was a real treat. Mr. Gildy, the mailman, knew that Miss Irene was Grandaddy—or, rather, used to be Grandaddy—but his respect for my momma was so solid that he conducted a wonderful little drama involving his solicitude over the sudden loss of her father, and how he hated to deliver a letter addressed to the deceased and all. Momma was equally creative, pretending to not recognize Grandma's wild handwriting. Oh, it was a wonder!

Momma carried the letter in to Grandaddy and left the room real quick. She banged around in the kitchen to let us know that she was totally unconcerned. Grandaddy, however, plunked down on the porch swing and got paler by the minute. He was holding the letter by one corner and fanning himself with it. I got him a glass of tea and sat down on the floor and pretended to work a splinter out of my foot.

Halfway through the tea he said, "Sister, my wife is coming home."

I said, "Yessir." And we sat, breathing hard, him fanning and me picking at my foot.

The next few weeks were something to remember, even though—according to Momma—nothing out of the ordinary happened before, during, or after.

Miss Irene packed up and left, supposedly because she missed the North so bad in spite of all the wonderful friends she had made down here. She left me three linen hankies with an 'I' embroidered in the corners, and some gardenia powder. After she was gone, rumors that she was romantically entangled with some Yankee circulated, but only for a while.

Then, Grandaddy's death was discovered to be a total, cruel fabrication on the part of the north Georgia branch of the family just so they could get their hands on his land up near Toccoa. Grandaddy had actually been lying in a hospital all this time, in a coma, not knowing his own name or whereabouts. Momma said fortunately she could save the tombstone for later, as it hadn't been carved yet; then she drove up to fetch both the tombstone and Grandaddy, who miraculously recovered just from hearing his own daughter's voice on the phone!

When they got home, Grandaddy went right outside in his undershirt to mow the grass, despite our begging him to rest up from his terrible ordeal.

Two days later Grandma came in on a Trailways bus, skinny as a bone and more suntanned than any lady should ever get. She brought us seashells and postcards of lurid sunsets, along with a listless baby alligator that had been throwing up since they were outside Talladega.

We never knew, of course, what transpired between Grandma and Grandaddy, but in no time at all they were back fussing at each other like the old days, making life as ordinary as could be.

Once in a while we would get a letter from Irene, who was up in Minnesota. Lord knows how Momma got those letters mailed to us, but she did and the ladies from church and the Garden Club were just pleased as anything to know how well Irene was doing up there in that frozen wasteland with her sweetheart. Marriage had apparently been mentioned.

Bubba and Nina and I finally went back to school and wrote our essays on "What I did This Summer" as truthfully as possible. Bubba wrote about going fishing up at Lake Raburn (which he did); Nina wrote about learning how to sew pleats and make divinity (which she did); and I wrote about how I had practiced writing stories (which I did).

Rowdy and the Bees

by

Kenneth Morgan

I answered the knock on my door that Saturday morning, in early summer of 1955, and was somewhat surprised to see Daddy standing there. He didn't visit very often and was usually busy on his farm at this time of day.

"I need a little help down at the house, Kenneth," he said. "Bring your rifle and come with me. Bring that old big rifle, that thirty-aught-six."

"What do you want me to shoot?" I asked.

"I'll tell you on the way. Just get the gun and come on," he said.

My Daddy, Mose Morgan, was a self-sufficient man and seldom called on us grown children for anything. He had supported his mother and father and a younger brother and sister even though he had a family of his own to provide for. The word "can't" wasn't in his vocabulary, a fact that had made all of us mad at one time or another.

We cut through the pasture, instead of taking the road, and Daddy filled me in on his problem as we walked.

"My bees swarmed and settled on a limb in the old pine by the pasture gate," he finally said. "I can't shake them off in the bee gum because they're about twenty feet high."

The bee gum was the hive the old-timers made out of short sections of hollow black gum logs. Then a small notch was cut into the bottom of the hollow log where it joined the board to enable the bees to go in and out. The top was a board that could be taken on and off. Daddy was trying to hive them and take them back home.

As we neared the old pine tree, I could see a cluster of bees about the size of a basketball hanging on the limb. When a young queen bee is ready to leave the old hive and start a new hive of her own, she gathers the drones and workers around her in a cluster until she is ready to leave.

"We don't have very much time," Daddy said. "They're just about ready to leave. I've got the gum set under the bees exactly where they'll fall into it when you shoot the limb off. I've already got a spot picked out on the limb where I want you to shoot, and I'll guarantee you they'll fall in the gum."

As I circled the tree with my gun, Daddy's little feisty squirrel dog, Rowdy, joined us, looking up in the tree and barking.

"Now, Rowdy," Daddy scolded, "you ain't got no business out here. You'll just be in the way." Daddy put Rowdy back in the yard, shut the gate, and told him in a stern voice, "Now, you stay in there."

Daddy's bees were the very ill-tempered little black bees native to East Texas, and when he got back I had a question for him. "What's gonna stop them bees from eatin' me up when I shoot them out?"

"I know you're afraid of them, Kenneth," he replied, "but you can get over behind that old log out there and they'll never see you. Besides, I'm gonna have the bee gum lid in my hand, and just as soon as they fall in I'm gonna cap 'em off."

I got settled in behind the log and raised the rifle to get sighted in on the limb. Just as he'd said, Daddy had his bee gum lid in hand and told me he was ready when I was. Rowdy was running back and forth inside the yard fence, whining and barking, and wanting to help us with whatever it was we were doing.

I could tell when I raised the rifle that Rowdy's excitement had reached a fever pitch. When the rifle roared, I caught sight of him out of the corner of my eye. He was sailing over the top of the fence.

If the bees had fallen directly after I fired the shot, Daddy might have reached the gum ahead of Rowdy. But the limb sagged and held momentarily before it fell. And I suppose another factor in the situation was that Rowdy was faster than Daddy was. Anyway, Rowdy reached the bee gum a fraction of a second before Daddy did and went in head first to retrieve the game.

"Git your tail out of there," Daddy yelled as he tried to pull Rowdy out with one hand and hold the lid in the other. After a few seconds of hard scuffling, he said, "If you like it so good, just stay in there. I'm gonna cap off this gum."

He had just popped the lid on when Rowdy had a quick change of heart. From my hiding hole I watched Daddy struggle with that lid.

Daddy was a strong man, but Rowdy still came out, bringing ninety-nine percent of those mad little black bees with him. They couldn't all fit on Rowdy, but they were so mad they had to get on something and sting it. That something was my daddy.

He was wearing a new felt hat and he pretty near wore it out. The bees flitted all over the place while Daddy swung and swung and swung. I was about to try to swat at some myself when Daddy gave it up and ran out of sight toward the banks of Hurricane Branch.

Rowdy tore out too, alternating between running and sliding on his back end. He would sit down flat on the ground with his hind feet sticking up in the air and use his front feet for propulsion. You'd be surprised how fast a dog can travel this way, when he's got a teacupful of bees under his tail.

I couldn't catch up with Daddy, but I could easily keep him located. He sounded like a herd of cape buffalo running through a dry canebreak.

When everything got quiet, I searched around and found him sitting on a log with his eyes swollen almost shut and his brand new hat in tatters.

"Do you want me to follow them bees, Daddy?" I asked. "They might settle down and we can try to hive them again."

This determined man, who had spent a lifetime never saying "can't," finally decided to give it a try. "No, son," he replied, not looking at me but watching Rowdy coming toward us now. "Let's just let them little S.O.B.s go."

The Gardener

by

Marjorie Rommel

I was twelve and my brother Frank was ten that Iowa summer Ma
sent us to borrow Mrs. McCready's wash boiler. It was hot and
still, and neither of us boys wanted to leave the coolness of the
root cellar, but Ma said go, so we went.

Alice McCready was a peppery, gospel-spouting widow in her
late seventies, scrawny and speckled as an old Buff Orpington
hen. Frank and I had never been inside her house, but we knew
where it was. Also we'd seen enough of her at church socials to
know we didn't like her any more than she liked us.

"Rapscallions!" She'd thrown the word at us as if it were a
hatchet when, only a few weeks before, she'd caught us transplant-
ing a wasp's nest into the hole beneath her outhouse,

It was two miles to Mrs. McCready's place, a long way in that
midsummer heat. We complained steadily every step of the first
mile. After that we were too busy just sweating and breathing.

The sun was high overhead, and our shadows were very
short when we turned down McCready Lane. Frank had begun to
whine he was thirsty, but I shushed him with the promise of a dip
in the old lady's horse tub. I pulled out my secret pouch of Bull
Durham, tucked a pinch under my lip and gave Frank a half
pinch to keep him quiet.

The heat was oppressive, the air humid and heavy. The stillness in the lane was so complete we could hear our hearts beating and the air going in and out of our chests. Our bare feet made soft flat sounds in the fine gray dust. Even the various buzzings of insects in the rose hedge that lined the lane were distinguishable.

By the time we reached the yard, we were almost dizzy with the heavy scent of Mrs. McCready's roses, intensified somehow by the heat.

There was no sign of anyone around the place and the house itself seemed deserted, though the parlor shades were up and the geraniums were set to air in a damp spot on the front steps.

Frank had a good grip on my belt loops even before we stepped onto the musty-smelling porch. I couldn't have backed up a step without knocking him down. "Scaredy-cat," I taunted him. "Think she's still mad about those wasps?"

My rap on the door was louder than I intended—a dull sound that the silence swallowed up without a trace—but no one answered. Frank and I stared at each other and waited. I remember that I could see the whites of his eyes all around their terrified centers. I'd gotten away, but she'd rapped him good about those wasps.

I'll admit now that I wanted to leave as passionately as my brother did, but I knew Ma would send us back if we came home without the wash boiler. We went around back to try the kitchen door, but got no answer. A slender green garter snake slithered away into the shade under the steps.

We decided to look for the wash boiler ourselves and started toward a weathered shed out back of the house.

As we approached, we became aware of a small, distinct snipping sound. Following it, we rounded the rose hedge where we found an old man carefully choosing roses to cut off from the hedge with a pair of pruning shears.

Frank's hand was like a vise on my belt loop, but I jerked him forward impatiently. We walked up to the gray-haired man.

"Afternoon, sir," I said, using my best manners. "We're here to see Mrs. McCready about the wash boiler."

He stopped working, fumbled for tobacco and papers in the pocket of his blue chambray shirt. Seen in profile, his face seemed petulant, angry. But front on, it was arresting—lined with a bitterness as deep and unforgettable as the smell of burnt almonds.

His ears were long, close to his head and intricately whorled. The iron-gray hair above them was dented from the band of a hat or cap he must have removed only moments ago. As he scrounged in his shirt pocket, I realized, with the nausea that so often attends fascinated shock, that the thumb and first finger were missing from his left hand.

The man was no one we had ever seen—a good trick in a town the size of Five Corners. Like a thousand other old men in those parts, he wore a shapeless gray knit vest in spite of the heat and his black Frisco jeans were pegged off logger-style at the top of his boots.

"You work for Mrs. McCready?" I persisted.

For a long moment, the old man considered us, then picked up his shears and went back to cutting roses—variegated pink and red ones he laid in a careful pile among the weeds.

Frank was shivering behind me and sweat—cold sweat—was pouring down my own sides. Frank had been scared since we hit the porch, and I—at least my body—was scared stiff too for some reason I couldn't understand. But I was indignant. Age, I thought, was no excuse for rudeness. And I didn't want to make another trip after that wash boiler. Not in this heat.

"Sir," I said firmly, "Mrs. McCready appears to be gone and our Ma needs to borrow her wash boiler. Can you tell us where it is?"

Finally the man jerked his mutilated hand toward the side of the house and stooped to retrieve his hat, hidden among the weeds. He picked up the roses he'd clipped, then turned down the hedgerow and disappeared. We followed, but found the shed empty.

Apart from that hedge, there was no cover of any kind—not

166

even tall grass—in Mrs. McCready's flat, weedy yard. Where had he gone?

We found the wash boiler hanging on a rusty nail under the eaves and, each taking an end, we trundled it home.

The shadows were slanting and it had cooled off some by the time we got home. Ma had been waiting and she scolded us for taking so long. We told her about the ornery old man by way of defense.

"Nonsense," she scoffed. "There's no man of *any* age on Alice McCready's patch."

When Father came home, Ma related our tale to him, expecting him to be amused, but he was not. Instead he pressed us for details of the man we had seen. As we told him, he frowned.

We'd apparently seen Case Johnston, a hard-drinking, bad-tempered old bachelor who squatted on the Daley place near town when Father was a boy. Johnston had been dead for years. No one even thought of him anymore.

It was highly unlikely that we could have heard such a detailed description from anybody else, Father mused, but why would Case Johnston haunt Alice McCready's place?

Father brooded through supper and after the dishes were done—Ma slamming the pots and pans to register her disapproval—he piled us all into the buckboard to return the borrowed wash boiler and possibly shed light on the mysterious gardener.

It was near first dark—crickets crying in the rose hedge, its perfume heavy as a funeral—when we reached the McCready place. Still there was no one home.

Father prowled around the house, found a lantern and went inside the shed. From a distance, he looked like an errant firefly. He came out again, his face grim with purpose in the lamp light, and returned to the house, taking the front steps at a single leap and forcing the door.

Inside, in the dark kitchen, Alice McCready was slumped over the table, dead. She was still wearing the leather house slippers and a holey, brown wool cardigan she'd adopted when her husband died. On the yellow oilcloth beside her astonished ex-

167

pression and scrawny, outstretched hand lay a bouquet of fresh-cut roses.

Ma stayed with the body while Father took us boys after Dr. James, who'd been alive long enough to know most of Five Corners' secrets. On the return trip, Father told him what we boys had seen.

The doctor was quiet for several miles, a pinched, far-away look on his usually peaceful face. His long, clean hands were folded in a kind of cross over the broken latch of his black bag. Then he began telling us about Case Johnston. How he'd loved Alice McCready for years, but she'd sworn to be true to her husband's memory and wouldn't accept him.

Case never married. He'd been happy just to be near Alice, the doctor said, coaxing those red and pink roses out of the Iowa dust, doing a little yard work for her now and then—or so it seemed. But he'd drunk himself to death in that little slant-roofed shed out back of Alice McCready's place more than twenty years before.

And the strangest thing about it: the hedge roses hadn't bloomed since he died.

Washing Daddy's Car

by

Irl Mowery

Taking my place at the observation window of the automated car wash, ready to root for my wife's convertible as it braves the gauntlet of steam and suds and whirling brushes, I remember my boyhood and the Saturday ritual of helping my father wash the car.

One of my father's unwritten rules was always to drive a clean car to church on Sunday. As my father used his car in the business of selling milking machines to farmers, by Saturday his fenders were caked with gumbo, the black mud of the coastal plains. For my younger brother and me, the high point of the week was Saturday afternoon, when we reveled in the messy camaraderie of washing the Pontiac with our dad.

These early memories of my father involve the cars he drove. When we still lived in the country, he drove a Model-T. Before my feet could reach the pedals, Daddy taught me when to push the lever underneath the steering wheel and advance the buzzing spark while he crouched in front and cranked her up. On Saturdays, when he drove us into town to get haircuts and see Rin-Tin-Tin at the picture show, we loved to play with the teat-cup rubbers that bounced around in the back seat.

After we moved into the city, where we had a cement driveway and no longer depended upon a windmill for water, Daddy drove a Model-A with a self-starter and I began to hold the hose while he washed. By the time he upgraded to the Pontiac, my brother got into the act.

When we were about eight and ten, we could hardly wait until Daddy finished his paperwork on Saturday mornings. As soon as he got home from the office, we would all three struggle into scratchy wool bathing suits, attach the hose, and prepare for the miracle of the chamois. We never tired of watching the thin beige pelt, dried stiff in the shape of the bucket where Daddy had draped it the previous week, melt in cold water and become a slippery blob.

Daddy would begin by laying the Pontiac's floor mats on the cement in front of the garage and Brother and I would take turns squirting the hose while he scrubbed them with a stubby broom. After hanging the mats over the fence to drip, Daddy aimed the hose as Brother and I took turns scrubbing the hub caps and the varnished wooden wheel spokes. Daddy then used his thumb to jet water from the hose and dislodge the gumbo under his fenders.

Next came my turn. I washed the roof, which my brother could not quite reach, by standing on the running board and wielding a ragged bath towel while Daddy held the hose. Then it was Brother's turn to massage the side and fenders while I aimed the hose. Next, Daddy washed the hood, careful not to slosh water onto the engine through the side vents. Then, with hose and brush, Daddy tackled the radiator, first the ornamental cap and then the front grill, always encrusted with squashed beetles and dragonflies.

Finally the chamois came into play to clean the windows and the windshield. After wringing out the chamois, Daddy used the thirsty pelt to sop up water from glass. Repeatedly twisting drab water out of the skin with powerful fists, he applied himself, rubbing in small circles until the glass gleamed. Our reward was being allowed to use the magical chamois to blot any drops of water remaining on the body. The chamois squeaked with delight.

After Daddy drove the shiny Pontiac into the garage, the real fun began. First he let us take turns sluicing mud and gravel off the cement. Then he turned the hose into a geyser, through

170

which we dashed back and forth, whooping with glee. Most fun of
all was the finale, in which Daddy let us turn the hose on him
until the skirt of his bathing suit was so sopping that it sagged halfway down his thighs.

Not until we unbuttoned the shoulder straps of our suits
and peeled them off in the privacy of the service porch did
Brother and I realize that our fingertips were shriveled blue and
we were shivering from cold hydrant water and delirium. After
toweling off and slipping into freshly ironed coveralls, we assem-
bled in the kitchen for peanut butter sandwiches on brown
bread, washed down with whole milk that left white moustaches
on our upper lips.

All those memories!

And now, at the car wash, my wife's convertible draws even
with my observation post opposite the hot wax machine. I tense
until the spigots jerk upward and spare the canvas top from wax.
As I follow the progress of glittering wire wheels and gleaming
whitewalls through a forest of flapping felts toward the drying
people at the end, something, somehow, is missing in this high-
tech version.

Moonlight Mirage

by

John H. Lambe

"Don't," Jim Reardon pleaded with his partner. "Rafe, no. Don't do it! For the love of all you've lost, forget this wild urge."

Two men sat staring at the center of a beaten-up slanted table in their weathered and tumble-down cabin. The objects of contention were two small bags of fine gold dust. The bags represented three weeks of unrelenting work, wrested from their claim up the hill, beyond the cabin's door.

Beside the bags sat a tallow candle, casting its flickering light dimly upon the walls. The light shimmered and danced, lending a ghostly vision to the old room and its occupants. The cabin's history contained many such men and probably many other confrontations much like the present one.

The area for miles around was the location of numerous deposits of "pocket gold." Two years ago a man stood a good chance of reaping huge profits from this kind of work. But the larger pockets had played out months ago and the remaining smaller ones required hours of back-breaking work to filter the soft grains of gold that were left in the ground. Rafe Benson and Jim Reardon were partners on a claim that yielded marginal amounts of gold, enough to keep their stomachs full and once in a while a debauch for Rafe. Reardon tried valiantly, and usually in vain, to keep Rafe from throwing his patiently acquired stock of mineral to the gin mills of town.

Rafe's arm reached out slowly, creeping to the buckskin bag. The powerful arm's coat-clad shadow was reflected by the single candle, jerking and wavering against the far wall. Reardon pleaded with his eyes, beseeching his long-time partner not to carry out his misguided scheme.

"Rafe," declared Jim, real pain in his voice, "it won't bring *her* any closer. Nothin' can do that."

At the mention of *her,* Benson's hand flashed to the gold and he clasped the bag tightly to his chest. Through gritted teeth he said, "You don't know...you never lived through the hell of losing them. Keep *her* out of this!"

Reardon knew he'd lost. He felt a shiver run the length of his back as the night wind moaned in the sagging rafters over their heads. He saw the bitter memories fill Rafe's mind as the shaggy miner's eyes fogged with an ancient love—a love gone long, long ago.

Benson suddenly jumped to his feet, the chair falling behind him, the sound ringing in the small room like a thunderbolt.

"I will go, Jim. You know it's got to be. A few more days and even you won't be able to live with me. I'll be back before sunrise, old friend." A tender gleam came into the eyes of the huge, ex-blacksmith miner. The trail of these two covered many a league and often Reardon had simply carried Rafe and his troubles on his own ample back. Rafe well knew the debt he owed his old friend and could hold no grudge against him.

Reardon's taut body fell back in the creaking chair. The emotional battle left him drained and he closed his eyes in defeat. He heard the shuffling steps reach the rough door, hung on leather hinges. The boards scraped as Rafe pulled on the latch. A random wind blew fresh air into the closed room, refreshing Jim with its coolness. He once again opened his eyes, but his friend was gone.

Rafe stepped into the roadway. Just appearing over the eastern mountains was a huge ripe moon. The honey-gold light bathed

173

the bowl containing the settlement in a glow from another world. Rafe could no longer contain his thoughts; they captured his mind as he strode determinedly toward his bottle of oblivion.

It seemed a lifetime ago when Rafe and Jim Reardon roamed the deserts of Arizona, California, and northern Mexico. Always searching for the elusive gold, they had only small grains of the gold dust to show for the barren leagues they had crossed. Yet, ever they hoped and wandered from one water hole to the next.

While buying supplies one day in a little town located in the foothills skirting the desert—below vast snow-clad peaks—Rafe caught a glimpse of a golden-haired young beauty. His future wife.

Turning to Jim, he made his declaration, "Old partner, I've come far enough. This will be my home. If you want to stay, why, you're welcome...or I'll give you my stake if you want to go back out there alone."

Rafe Benson married the most beautiful girl in Arizona. Her blue eyes shone clear, piercing his heart with the love she carried for him. Her hair was the exact color of the radiant moon over his head. He loved the girl with every fiber of being he possessed.

Two weeks later, Jim, now alone, again entered the domain of blasting sun and faraway shimmering mirage. Rafe remained, opened a forge, and became a well-respected member of the little community.

A short year later, as Reardon set out on his solitary quest, he left Rafe Benson wreathed in all the joys a man could possibly possess. Rafe's wife carried their child...their future. Happiness for the lovers could be no greater.

In the late fall, the leaves bathed the hardwoods in a crimson wash of color and Reardon wandered back into the tiny hill settlement exhausted. Expecting to see the mother and her new child, he found only a lonely, bitter, and defeated man.

When the full term came and the baby was ready to be born, Rafe could not find the doctor. His beloved wife developed complications delivering and he lost both mother and child. She screamed her life away in uttermost pain. In Rafe's mind, he caused their deaths through the clumsy uselessness of his huge and impotent hands.

174

He buried the two he loved most, mother and child, side by side, in a single rough pine box, their golden curls lying upon blanched waxen faces. He sold the house and boarded the smithy windows.

Jim found his long-time friend had taken to the bottle and was lying in a heap on the filthy floorboards of a half-rotted shack. Realizing the only possible cure, he scrubbed the ill-smelling hulk of his old companion, purchased new supplies including a case of whiskey to lure Rafe along like a recalcitrant burro, and dragged the poor unfortunate man back into the inferno of the winter desert far to the south.

At first Rafe blundered along stolidly following Jim, water hole to distant ridge. Weeks later, when the supply of liquor ran out, Benson began to reenter the world and take note of his surroundings. Too far from civilization to buy cheap whiskey, he was forced to live with himself and his horrible memories.

The naked red rock dancing in the afternoon heat came to dominate his mind and excluded the scalding visions of his past. His heat-seared mind slowly recovered. The nights of unsurpassed beauty when the new moon would rise and reveal a smoky world filled with the ancient beauty of distant pasts helped him to bury his loved ones in the peace they could not gain in life. The distant wavering blue mountains always seemed beyond their slowly creeping gait, but they lured them with promises of cold spring water in rippling streams.

Yet the cure never took. Each time the men encountered a village, Rafe fought the call of liquor, but he always succumbed to it in the end. But, thankfully, the spells were far apart and caused little harm.

Little did Jim suspect that a prolonged stay in a cabin near a town would lead to the fast deterioration of his friend. Never would he have consented to this journey into the California goldfields if he had known.

Since they settled in the old cabin and remained near the semi-civilized settlement of Raven Creek, Rafe had fallen hard back into the self-pity and recrimination that he had left far away in Arizona. Now, day by day, Jim planned how to force Rafe from the mountains and return to the cleansing desert.

The wind blew, falling and swirling from the mountain heights around Rafe. Picking up dirt and grit, the gust forced him to work his way downward. A small snow-melt creek, rambling from the rock crags high above, found its way into his boots as he forded it; the chill brought life back to his mind. Thoughts of the present quickened his pace to reach the companionship of the saloon and the peace of drink.

The ethereal night filled the valley and calmed his callow mind as he trudged onward. Nearing the outskirts of town, he passed the first secluded cabin. In passing he heard a tiny sound above the night wind. Halting in mid-stride, Rafe tilted his head to better hear the sound that haunted his memory.

It came again, floating from the cabin, faint on the wind. He turned and searched the dark shadows. A just-perceptible lighter space gave clue of the origins of what now sounded like a whimper. He moved silently to the spot.

He could make out the shimmering form of a small child. Could this be what reached out to him? Coming closer, he found, indeed, it was a child.

The giant miner, materializing out of the night, scared the child and she gasped before Rafe could reassure her of his peaceful intent.

"Honey, it's only old Rafe...Benson. It's little Polly Larson, ain't it? Polly." Rafe tried to modify his usually raspy, rumbling voice, "What's the trouble?"

"Oh, Mr. Benson, you scared me," whispered the little girl. Anyone would have been scared. The big man resembled nothing more than a bear shuffling from the fir and pine-clad mountain slopes. The smoky moonlight and cool wind showed the child's presence of mind—she didn't run screaming from him.

"Are you crying, child? Come, tell Rafe your friend. Is there something I can do?" Rafe and all the other local miners, loved the golden-haired girl that belonged to the clerk of the only mercantile store in the area. Ole Larson, his wife, and their only child, Polly, moved into the cabin that served as a home a year and a half ago. He worked for wages, hoping the town would solidify into a respectable community. The area came close to reminding him of his native Sweden. Their daughter was now a product of the rough goldfields. Any of the tough-edged men in the valley would have killed a full-grown grizzly, barehanded, for the child.

"It's Daddy, Mr. Benson." She stopped to sniffle, "He went away last Tuesday. Mother says we must leave…but, can't."

"Went? Went where, honey?" Rafe began to feel his temper rise that a man should leave a family such as this one of his own free will.

"He died. A terrible fever came last week. Mother said it was…oh, I don't know…and now he's just gone, forever." At the end, she couldn't carry on the thought. Tears rolled down her satin cheek.

Rafe reached out and took the tiny, fragile body and held her close to him. The child wept, burying her face on his broad and powerful chest. When the spell passed, she lifted her head back to look into Rafe's eyes. A tremor swept from deep within his chest as he realized he was gazing into the face of the little one he himself had lost long ago.

The feeling was almost more than Benson could bear. He reeled under the blow. The shock vibrated through him and sent waves of tenderness out his fingertips. The child felt his empathy and responded with the gentle look in her blue eyes that were reflecting the hazy light.

The wind, modified by the house before them, gently lifted the fine silken hair on her head and the soft gold of the moonlight created a halo about her. Rafe could only think of his lost child. Remembering, wishing, he gazed long moments at this wraith from the past.

Polly was continuing her explanation when Rafe came to his senses. "She says we cannot leave; we are poor and have no money. Grandfather is in Missouri, and that is across the whole world. Our food will only last a few more days, Mother says, but I think our friends will help us. Don't you think so, Mr. Benson?"

Rafe shook off the dreams running vehemently through his

head and answered her, "Of course, honey, we'll all help you. You want to go to your Grandpappy?" Rafe's hand flew to his heart. Under the filthy leather coat he found the heavy little buckskin bag and, holding her tiny white hand, he placed it in her keeping. "Here," he said.

"Oh," she cried. No one in the mountains would fail to recognize a gold pouch.

"Ssssh," Rafe held his finger up. "Don't wake your mom. Take it and in the morning give it to her. She'll know what to do." The tears were beginning to burn his own eyes now as he bid her good night.

From the dusky roadway, Rafe watched as Polly entered the cabin. He stood there with lowered head, deep in thoughts filled with the relentless memories. Finally he turned back up the mountain, broke and forced to live with dreadful dreams that he could not lose.

At the frigid creek crossing he halted, dreading to wet his feet yet again. As he pondered the night's happenings, a strong breeze filled his eyes with grit. When he had wiped them free, he saw the dark outline of a desperado facing him with the big bore of a pistol pointed steadily at his stomach.

"Awright, friend, take a pull at them stars," growled the bandit.

Putting his hands on high, Rafe chuckled and said, "You done missed out on this job—I'm broke."

"Broke!" The man cursed quietly and searched the burly miner. When the rough hands had finished, he hoarsely whispered, "So! You're poor as me. Well, I'll show you not to carry some dust, in case we meet agin'...." The big pistol came up in readiness to lash at the blacksmith.

For all his size, Rafe Benson was as quick as one of the tawny lions that roamed these mountains. His massive left fist ripped upward out of the darkness into the outlaw's stomach with huge effect. The man crumpled forward and Rafe's right fist slashed into his unprotected jaw. A hollow sound followed by a crack, as if something had quickly given way, greeted the glad ears of the miner.

The desperado, pistol flying, went rolling off the side of the trail into the creek. He recovered in the chilly water and fled into the brush. Rafe watched, hugely pleased with himself. Grinning, he looked down and saw the dull glint of the gun lying in the dust.

When he reached to recover the weapon, he noticed a much brighter gleam. The barrel of the pistol pointed directly at the shiny object. Picking it up between his strong fingers, Rafe saw it was a golden tooth, apparently from the outlaw's jaw. So, he had indeed done some lasting damage to the desperado.

"Well, the dirty...deserved what he got!" thought Rafe. Then the moon reflected a broad smile crossing his face. This was gold—and the saloon would accept any gold. That outlaw was going to buy him at least one drink!

Rafe turned immediately and retraced his steps. Shortly, he entered the Golden Bucket Saloon and was surrounded by the familiar sounds and smells. He looked the crowd over and saw many a familiar face. One man's eye caught his from the poker table.

"Rafe, over here. Come on an' join us," called Charlie Slack.

Rafe worked across the crowded room and sat in a vacant chair. "Howdy, Charlie. Cain't play, unless this here piece will buy me a hand." He laid the gold tooth on the table.

Charlie laughed at the bet, but allowed that it would do for one hand of twenty-one. Two cards flipped over the green felt and Rafe peeked at a pair of queens! Twenty. He won the hand and then parlayed the toothy stake to over fifty dollars. He pulled his winnings and quit the game. To gamblers in the gold country, fifty dollars was no more than a haircut, so they didn't think anything of his going for a bottle.

Rafe piled his little stake on the bar and ordered what it would purchase. The bartender surveyed the pitiful pile and set three bottles before the miner. Two for the gold and one for old times' sake. Rafe grabbed his prizes and kicked back the chair at an empty table, at long last to fulfill his quest.

Three hours later he stumbled out the swinging doors, headed for home. Scant feet from the saloon, he began to doubt whether he could reach the cabin or if it was even possible to find it!

Rounding a corner into a littered alley, he tripped over a rain barrel, careened off the wall of a building, and fell, full length, into a pile of trash.

"Well, danged if it don't feel like bed," thought Rafe and he passed quietly into unconsciousness.

Early, just after the sun rose over the eastern mountains, Polly and Mrs. Larson came hurrying down the wooden sidewalk. They hastened to catch the early Sunday stage headed into the sunrise and home.

Mrs. Larson talked rapidly to the girl, "We'll have everything when we reach father's house. Never will we have to put up with these foul, disreputable men. Oh," she spotted Rafe's feet protruding from the alleyway bed he occupied, "Polly, do come away from that…thing."

Polly glanced at the prostrate body as her mother pulled her along and away from the drunk. "Mother, I think…"

"Do come along, dear. We must hurry if we are not to miss this stage." They carried two cardboard suitcases and Polly struggled with a pillowcase stuffed with belongings. So it was not her fault she didn't fully recognize her lonely benefactor lying beside their road home.

And, truth to tell, Rafe would not have wanted to be seen. He was where he wanted to be—in blissful, undreaming sleep.

Grandmother Turner's New Life

by

Judith Bell

"You move slower than any thirteen-year-old I ever saw." Grandmother Turner shoved some cereal boxes toward Emogene's place at the table and gathered her pocketbook and keys. "Get on over here and eat something. I can't be late for my hair tint."

In the months since Grandaddy died, Grandmother had given up two things: cooking and staying home. She was in the full glory of what she called her retirement. All the relatives she had waited on for forty years were finally dead and she had taken to pleasuring herself with a vengeance. Emogene had spent every weekend since her grandfather's death with her grandmother. Saturday mornings they went to the beauty parlor, then had lunch at the drugstore. Sunday mornings they went to church.

At first, Emogene's mother had come too. But she claimed that "carting Mama all over the face of the earth" wore her out, and Grandmother decided that just because her husband had never let her learn to drive was no reason not to learn now. After a few Saturday mornings of practice in the church parking lot with her daughter, Grandmother sent her home, insisting she have Emogene each weekend for company.

181

"Do you think I need a new permanent wave, Emogene? My hair's not curling up like it was." Grandmother Turner paused to stare at her reflection in the toaster as she bent down to pour some milk on Emogene's cereal. "There's that revival at the church next week and I do want to look good for that. Well, I could never get it today; that Ruby keeps herself booked up tight as a nut. Maybe I'll just get me a new hat instead." Arms folded across the low shelf of her bosom, she stood by the table watching Emogene spoon up her cereal. "Eat a little more then come on out here to the piano," she said, moving into the hall. "Let's play a hymn before we leave."

Emogene dropped her spoon and was on her grandmother's heels, following her into the dim hallway that ran the length of the house. When Grandmother Turner played, she hit the keys with a sense of purpose. With the strike of each chord, the force of her intentions coursed through the knotted veins that rose and fell along the backs of her gnarled hands.

"Sing with me, Emogene. Singing frees the spirit," she said, playing the opening bars of her favorite hymn.

Emogene's voice was lost in the fullness of her grandmother's as they sang: "Shall We Gather at the River?"

Grandmother Turner spent all her free moments at the piano. In the middle of making biscuits or pie she would wipe her hands across the front of her apron and run into the hall to play just one more hymn before Grandaddy came in from the fields.

"Aurilla, leave off playing that thing," he would bellow before he was halfway in the back door. "I swear that's what you do all day while I'm out working." After his mother died he was never sure what Grandmother Turner had been up to and this worried him. He would go straight to the dining room table and sit, the strain of being indoors wearing on him while he waited for his supper to appear. Grandmother's lips would go tight, the color pressed out of them, as she closed the cover over the keys and rose to return to the kitchen.

Emogene remembered the day that his hold on her grandmother came to an end. The afternoon after his burial, Emogene sat in the parlor with her grandmother, the shades drawn against the cold air that seeped through the windows. Empty of mourners for the first time in days, the house was quiet, the only sound coming from their forks hitting their plates as they finished off the last of the lemon chiffon cake left by Mrs. Jenkins. A howling wind rushed down the chimney, chilling them as it swept through the house, slamming doors in its wake.

"Well, that was the Holy Ghost." Grandmother Turner pressed her finger against her plate to get the last of her cake crumbs. A clear sign that she had had enough of this mourning business, she got up and went in to her piano.

"That ought to do us for hymn-singing this morning." Grandmother Turner closed the cover. "Go on out and get the car windows rolled down, Emogene."

Emogene ran down the hall to the kitchen and out the back door. She opened the car windows all the way; Grandmother wouldn't mind the wind since they were going to the beauty parlor first thing. She left the doors open to let the seat covers cool off some and rocked back on her heels, waiting.

Grandmother Turner liked to take the back stairs one at a time, holding the bannister for good measure. "I'll not break my hip rushing," she would say. "Only trip I'll have then will be to the hospital."

"I want to eat at Walgreen's when we get done at the beauty parlor," Emogene said when her grandmother was on solid ground.

"Suits me fine." Grandmother Turner motioned for her to get into the car. "I wouldn't mind having me a cold plate, hot as it's going to be out today."

Ruby's Beauty Bungalow was in an old Esso station on the main road leading into Potter. Not one for parallel parking, Grandmother Turner favored Ruby's and her big parking lot over the beauty parlor in town. Most of the older women around Potter felt the same way. Inside Ruby's the chemical smells of dye and permanent waving fluid outlasted the perfume of shampoos and rinses.

Before going inside, Grandmother Turner usually gave

Emogene a dollar and sent her across the road to Craven's Store for Sugar Daddys and fireballs—candy hard enough to last through their morning at Ruby's—but today they were running late.

"Get on in the beauty parlor and tell Ruby I'm here, before she gives away my appointment," Grandmother Turner said before she had the car stopped. "Besides, I want to put on some lipstick before I make a public appearance."

Opening the frosted glass door Emogene heard the roar of hair dryers above the hiss of spray net cans and the hum of women talking. She wandered past the beauty operators to where Ruby was settling a customer under the hair dryer.

"Now Ruby, careful with that heat," the woman was saying. "I get a headache something awful when the ear pieces on my glasses heat up."

Ruby clucked sympathetically and turned the heat on high.

"Well, Emogene, are you here for the works today?" Ruby patted her blonde beehive, turning to give herself an admiring smile in the mirrored wall above the hair dryer.

"No, Ma'am. My grandmother says to tell you she'll be right in," Emogene answered.

"All right, honey." Ruby leaned over the coffee table where she kept her magazines. "Here's some picture books to keep you occupied."

Holding the magazines close, Emogene followed Ruby over to the chair across from her station. She sifted through the magazines, discarding the *Ladies' Home Journal.* The fashion magazines were Emogene's favorite part of her Saturday mornings here. Somewhere inside them was the secret to a different life. She could feel it move just beyond her fingertips as she turned the glossy rich-colored pages.

Grandmother Turner walked in the door. "Ruby, I want you to go easy on the blue in this hair tint."

"You're the one had your mind set on blue." Ruby snapped the pink plastic cape sharply in the air. "Let's go get you rinsed out." Ruby patted Emogene's knee. "We'll be right back."

Emogene hardly noticed them. She was already lost in her

magazine in which tall, graceful women wore elegant clothes in exotic places. Here they were in Egypt by the pyramids, looking cool as ice in long, flowing robes, the desert sun making their faces shine like gold.

Grandmother Turner settled into Ruby's chair.

"Let's go to Egypt sometime," Emogene said.

"Hee, hee, Egypt, huh?" Grandmother Turner paused, watching Emogene in Ruby's big mirror. "Careful you don't tell your mother about that. She'll be on me again for feeding your big ideas," she said. "Let me see what you're looking at."

Emogene leaned forward, holding the magazine close to her grandmother's face.

"Those gals'll be burned to a crisp wearing such as that in the desert. Maybe we will go to Egypt," Grandmother Turner said. "Catch me some rich sheik, right, Ruby?"

"What you want some sheik bossing you around for, Miz Turner?" Ruby shook her head as she combed blue dye through Grandmother Turner's hair.

Grandmother Turner sniffed. "I don't suppose they're any worse than men anywhere else."

"Well, I hate to be the one to remind you," Ruby began, although Emogene could see she didn't mind at all, "but to hear you tell it, you already had one man telling you what to do and that was one too many."

Grandmother Turner's mouth went all tight, and in her mind Emogene saw her closing the piano, going into the kitchen to wait on Grandaddy.

The Longest Summer

by

Beth S. Moore

"Nisha," I whispered, "lie still!"

The big dog twitched in her sleep. The weight of my legs on her back wasn't enough to wake her, but probably kept her from sleeping soundly.

Still, the sun's heat and the warmth of her body eased the pain in my legs. I'd been sick for several months with rheumatic fever; the doctor feared heart damage. I was recovering, but my weak legs still hurt. My tenth birthday would be in a month and I wanted to walk by then.

Moving restlessly, I woke the dog. Nisha turned her big head and perked her ears up as if asking what was wrong. I smiled and reached to pet her. How her doggy smell comforted me, that faint animal smell that made Mom wrinkle up her nose. I liked it.

I moved my legs off the dog. "Go, Nisha, go get Mom," I said, pointing to our big, old farmhouse. She jumped up and ran, barking all the way to the back door.

Perspiration beaded on my forehead and I needed to move out of the unseasonably hot, June sun. The backyard sloped gently down to huge, leafed-out cottonwood trees that followed the fence line, but the shade no longer reached my spot of grass.

"My stars, I hear you, Nisha," I heard Mom say. "I'm com-

186

ing!" Hearing her name, Nisha waved her fluffy tail. Mom laughed and stooped to pet her. Then my mother moved her arms under mine and slid me over the slick grass toward the cottonwoods. Soon the shade covered me, and I stretched on the grass, seeking a comfortable spot.

Once still, the dog lay by me, and I gave her a hug. Then I held her so she wouldn't lick my face. "Down, you silly dog. Don't you know you stink?"

Nisha stretched to lick my face again because she knew my tone was teasing. "Why do dogs like to lick so much, Mom?"

"That's their way of kissing and telling you they love you, I guess," said Mom. "Nisha, down." When Nisha obeyed, Mom put my legs back over the dog's back. "Dad'll help you practice walking later this afternoon, Rachel."

"Will I walk by my birthday?" I asked.

"That's a whole month away, but with Nisha's help, lots of prayers, and the hot sun, we just might make it," my mother said as she fluffed my long hair out on the pillow, bent and kissed me, and walked back to the house.

Nisha's whimper drew my attention back to her, and she wagged her tail. Her ears perked up the way they did when she wanted an answer to a question.

"It's okay, old girl. Go to sleep," I reassured her. A gentle wag of her tail answered me. Then she put her nose on her paws and did just that.

A bee buzzing from the tulips to the heavily laden lilac bush caught my attention and I inhaled deeply. It was a smell as sweet as the taste of honey itself. The noisy caw of blackbirds out in the fields where Dad was plowing blended with the sound of the bees. In my mind I could visualize the birds swarming over the fresh-turned earth snatching up the insects Dad would be uncovering. In contrast to the shrill caws came the meadow lark trilling her sweet melody over and over. Soon I, too, was lulled to sleep.

"Wake up, Rachel," came Dad's deep voice. "Time for a little walking practice."

I rubbed my eyes and noted the lengthening shadows. Strong arms pulled me to my feet and held me tight. I marvelled at how I had to consciously put one foot in front of the other, but with Dad there, I could do it!

"Look at Nisha," Dad said, "she really thinks she's helping."

Nisha had grabbed the edge of my dress and lifted her head high. She was wagging her big, fluffy tail constantly. When we laughed, the dog dropped my dress to bark at us.

"You're getting so much stronger." Dad reached down and petted Nisha. "Enough for today. Let's go in and eat supper."

Once we'd eaten, Mom soon had me ready for bed. I read until I felt sleepy. As I reached down to the side of my bed to give Nisha her good night hug, I heard Dad's voice.

"I've been so afraid, Amanda," he said.

"I know, I know. I have, too," Mom said. "But I'm sure Rachel's well on the road to recovery now."

I could hear Dad's sigh clear in my room. "If only she doesn't have heart damage."

"She won't, John, she won't," Mom answered.

I snuggled down in the covers and my lids drooped. Strange, I thought. I'd known Dad had been afraid, but I'd never guessed Mom had been, too.

The month went by fast after all, and I was walking alone. Not for too long or very far, but I could walk!

That ten-year-old birthday was one I'll never forget. My cousins, my brothers, and I had such fun. But once all the people had gone home, my legs seemed so weak and shaky that I longed for bed. Mom brushed my hair back from my face with her cool, gentle hands. "I'm afraid we've let you overdo it."

I looked around for Nisha, suddenly aware I hadn't seen her for some time.

"Nisha," I called. "Here, Nisha, here, Nisha!"

But she didn't come. Anguished, I called her name over and over, pleading desperately as tears filled my eyes.

"Nisha, oh, Nisha, please come!" I cried.

"Rachel," comforted Dad, "go in the house with Mom. The boys and I will hunt for her. She must be close. Probably took out after a rabbit."

Groping toward the house, I'd have fallen if Dad hadn't

caught me. He carried me into the house, sat me down, and hurried out to begin the search.

Mom and I looked at each other in silent sorrow. We both knew Nisha never strayed. How could I have been so busy with the excitement of the party that I had forgotten her? In my anxiety, I could feel the fluttering beat of my heart. We sat in the encroaching darkness, waiting.

Finally the door slammed, startling us both. Dad flipped on the lights and I knew they hadn't found her. How could such a beautiful birthday have ended so dreadfully?

Long days passed without a sign of Nisha. I had trouble sleeping and no food tempted me. It took an effort to do my exercises with Dad. Everything reminded me of her. I relived the moments when I'd hugged Nisha, holding her close, burying my arms in her thick fur. I remembered the doggy smell that had always comforted me and the feel of her wet, rough tongue. Sharp pain at my loss never left me and tears were always welling in my eyes.

One morning, over a week later, my father's deep voice downstairs woke me. "Amanda," he told Mom, "several dogs have turned up missing since the night of Rachel's party. And they're all dogs that would make good sheep dogs. It was rotten luck the thieves happened to come through on Rachel's birthday, because any other time, Nisha would have been with her."

I jumped out of bed and took the stairs as fast as my weak legs could move. Once in the kitchen, I threw myself at Dad. "You've found Nisha. Oh, Dad, you've found Nisha!"

"Whoa, Rachel, I don't know for sure. There's a chance, though, that Nisha's on some grassy, pine-covered mountain right now. Can't you imagine her nipping at sheep's heels to keep them under control? She's probably having a wonderful time with all that space to roam in."

I shook my head frantically, "Not without me!" My voice rose to a scream. "We must go get her. I'll hurry and get dressed."

I turned to leave, but Dad caught me.

"Wait, Rachel," Dad said. "I have no idea who might have

taken her or where she might be. These Big Horn Mountains are far too vast for us to go chasing all over them."

I couldn't believe it. I stared at Dad. "You mean we're not going after Nisha?" Tears wet my cheeks and fell onto my gown, soaking it. Dad pulled me onto his lap and wiped my face.

"We couldn't hope to find her now, but those men come back in the fall and, as each man brings in his herd of sheep, I promise I'll be there watching. If that's what happened to Nisha we'll find her. In the meantime, Mr. Murphy's German Shepherd just had a new batch of pups and he said we could have one."

I shook my head in horror. How could Dad mention such a thing? "I don't ever want another dog." My eyes met Dad's. "You don't think we'll ever find Nisha, do you?"

His glance never flinched. "There's a chance something else happened and you mustn't get your hopes too high. But we could sure use another dog around here; Nisha was always with you."

I stared at Dad. I knew he thought another dog would help get my mind off Nisha. Well, it wouldn't work.

"No," I said, swallowing hard over the lump in my throat.

Dad shrugged and ruffled my hair. "Go wash up and comb that yellow mop of yours and let's eat."

That very afternoon Dad came home carrying the cutest, blackest, littlest pup I'd ever seen. "Mr. Murphy has a lot of people already wanting this dog, so I thought I'd better take her," he said.

He set the puppy down and it ran to me. It began licking my bare feet and falling over itself as it tumbled around me. My arms ached to pick her up. I could almost feel her wiggling body close to mine and smell her puppy smell. But I didn't, because somehow I felt if I loved another dog, I'd never find Nisha.

"I'm sorry, Dad, but I just don't want her," I said.

He put his arms around me. "I know, Rachel, but you can love this puppy without forgetting Nisha."

My brothers came running up just then and the puppy hurried toward them, her little body twisting and turning with delight. I ran into the house trying not to hear the sound of her yippy little barks. Once in the house though, I walked to the window and watched.

The shrill voice of my brother, Andrew, came through the open door. "Can we keep her, Dad, can we? Nisha was always Rachel's dog and that wasn't fair."

"Yes," answered Dad. "I've got to have a dog around here. It won't hurt us to have two even if we do find Nisha. I'd hoped Rachel would take to the puppy though."

Then my youngest brother, Sam, spoke up, "I'm glad she didn't. Let's name her Licorice."

I turned in disgust. What a dumb name. I knew I could have thought of a better one. Still, I resolutely picked up a book to read. I tried to shut my mind to all thoughts of the puppy.

The summer dragged on. I avoided the little black puppy. Whenever I did see her, she would sit down on her little haunches and cock her head to one side with a little bark. She seemed to be asking me why I didn't like her.

Fall came at last and Dad came in one night full of excitement.

I grabbed his hand, certain I knew what had happened. "Are the sheepherders in yet, Dad? Have you found Nisha?"

He swallowed and made an effort to speak calmly. "All the wagons aren't in yet, Rachel, but the families who lost dogs are watching. It'll snow soon, so it won't be long now before the rest come in. Those sheepherders don't like winter in the mountains."

"But, Dad," I started to say. He didn't want to meet my eyes and I sensed he was hiding something from me.

"No more questions, Rachel. I told you I'd let you know if Nisha is with any of the sheepherders," he said.

His tone silenced me, but I wasn't content. I couldn't go to sleep and once the house was quiet, I heard my parents talking. I crept down the hall toward the kitchen. Their voices were soft and I strained to hear.

"I've found Nisha, Amanda," Dad said, "but I don't know what to do."

Shock kept me quiet. Found Nisha, and he didn't know what to do? What did he mean?

"Old Mac McIntosh has her," he continued. "I guess he stole

191

Nisha. Officer Murphy told me." I remembered talk about McIntosh, an old Scotsman whose wife and children were killed in a
fire years ago. He'd been strange ever since. He'd just lived with
his sheep and his dog. Then his dog died.

Dad's voice sounded funny, sort of soft and sad. He stopped
talking for a minute and I wanted to rush into the room. But
something held me back.

"I hurried up to his camp knowing how happy Rachel would
be," Dad said. "The old man cried the minute he saw me. Tears
rolled down those weathered old cheeks, startling me so. Then
he said he was sorry that he'd stolen my dog, but he'd just had to
have one so that he could bear the loneliness."

Dad's voice sounded like he might be crying, too. I could
hear him blow his nose, then he went on. "There's no doubt he
loves Nisha and Nisha loves him. Not in the same way she loves
Rachel, I'm sure. But she certainly didn't want to come with me. I
called her and she'd start to come. Then she'd whine and look
back at the old man sitting there with tears running down his old,
whiskered face. I wanted to surprise Rachel, but now I don't know
what to do! How can I take the dog away from him? Licorice is
going to be a good ranch dog, but that won't matter to Rachel.
What shall I tell her?"

"The truth, John," I heard Mom say. "She might find out
some day and she'd lose faith in you."

My heart started beating in agitation. The doctor had told
my parents I shouldn't get excited, but I couldn't believe what I'd
heard. Some old man had stolen my dog and now my own dad
wanted to let him keep her. I forgot the feelings of pity I'd started
to feel. This was my Nisha he was talking about. I stumbled into
the kitchen.

"Dad, Nisha is mine. I'd never have walked again without
her. You know that! You can't mean you'd let an old man who
stole her just keep her? He has no right, no right!" I started to
shake.

Dad hugged me as I collapsed in his arms. "I know, Rachel, I
know I had to tell you. I told McIntosh we'd be there tomorrow
to pick Nisha up. But Rachel, this old man has no one."

192

"I know," I interrupted. "He lost his wife and children in a fire, but that doesn't give him the right to steal my dog!"

The room became so quiet I could hear my heart beating fast. I couldn't meet either one of my parents' eyes knowing I'd see disappointment in them. But I didn't care!

Dad sighed and his soft voice conveyed his sadness. "I told him we'd be there tomorrow. So go to bed, Rachel."

I turned and walked back to my room. I did feel sorry for the old man, even though it hadn't sounded like it. But Nisha was my dog and he had to give her to me. I'd missed her so, but tomorrow we'd be together again.

I tossed and turned, unable to sleep. My mind kept flashing pictures of Nisha and this reminded me of the day that Mom had cut my hair. When Nisha had seen my yellow hair falling on the ground, she'd pulled at Mom's skirts and jumped up and down barking. Neither Mom nor I could figure out what was wrong with her. Then she'd sniffed at my hair on the ground and finally she put her head back and howled.

"My stars," Mom had said, "I believe Nisha thinks I'm hurting you and she doesn't know what to do."

Then I'd pretended to cry as Mom snipped my hair and Nisha went crazy, barking and running around us. Mom had laughed until she cried, telling me to stop.

Eventually good thoughts of Nisha lulled me to sleep.

The next morning, I hurried Dad until he spoke crossly. "Rachel, you'll have your dog. Now calm down and leave me alone until I'm ready to go."

I subsided, knowing he wasn't angry with me. He just didn't want to take Nisha away from the old man. I felt sorry, too, but I knew all I wanted was my arms around my big, old, shaggy dog again.

Finally Dad announced he was ready. Once we were loaded in the car and on our way, I kept quiet. The winding road looked like a ribbon up the mountainside. As the old car sputtered in protest, I felt that even the car didn't approve of what I was doing. *But I don't care if anybody agrees,* I thought, as I flipped my hair over my shoulder and tried to relax my rigid body.

At last Dad pulled into a tree-filled cove, and the beauty of the pines clustered next to a grassy meadow calmed me. Once out of the car Dad and I found a little path. Nisha's barking reached us just as the sight of an old battered pickup, perched on two flat tires, parked by a covered wagon came into view. Abandoned tin cans and loose papers marred the scene, and I resented the intrusion of such junk in the beautiful mountains.

"This is his home?" I whispered in disgust.

Dad frowned and nodded his head. He reached to knock on the splintered door of the shabby wagon. I heard a gruff voice say, "Come in."

I stumbled up the steps and Dad reached around to me to open the door. After the bright sunshine, I couldn't see at first in the dim light of the small wagon. Then I saw Nisha sitting at the old man's feet. Unbearable excitement made me tremble.

"Nisha," I cried, holding out my arms.

She wagged her tail and I knew her eyes recognized me, but she didn't come! I couldn't believe it. Even though my attention focused on the dog, bad smells crowded in on me. The odor of burned bacon mingling with strong tobacco was soon overpowered by the reek of an unwashed body and an unkempt dog. I had to swallow hard to keep from throwing up.

Rusted pans full of dried-out food were piled on the tiny cooking stove, with broken dishes on a box that must be his table. I imagined I could see bedbugs crawling on the tumbled, dirty bed where the old man sat. I didn't want to touch anything, that is, except Nisha. The loud ticking of a battered alarm clock found an echo in my damaged heart.

"Nisha," I begged. "Don't you know me? Come here. Please, Nisha, come to me!"

Her tail wagged frantically and she barked a welcome. Yet no matter how I called and entreated, she wouldn't leave the old man's side. I trembled with indignation. What was the matter with her? I reached out and grabbed the collar on her neck. The collar I'd put there myself.

"Come, girl," I pleaded, leaning closer to her.

Nisha licked my hand and wagged her tail constantly, but

194

she didn't make any effort to move. Anger tensed my body and then I met McIntosh's bleary, blue eyes. That was a mistake. Eyes so lonely and hurt, and so full of tears that they trickled down his smudged, wrinkled cheeks. I felt my own eyes fill.

"Go, girl," the old man whispered, "go with Rachel."

His voice cracked and I knew he'd swallowed a sob. Nisha stood up and pulled away from my hand. She put her front paws on the old man's knees and looked into his face, licking his tears. He put his arms around her and hugged her tight. Then he released her and stood up. He took a grimy handkerchief out of his pocket, blew his nose, and repeated, "Go, girl!"

Nisha looked at him and then moved toward me as I backed out of the tiny wagon. Dad stood waiting for me. But once the dog reached the step, she sat down and looked back at the old man. I could hardly swallow over the painful lump in my throat, and tears stung my eyes. Hurt had replaced the anger I'd felt. I hadn't been angry since I'd looked into those old eyes.

"Nisha," I begged, "don't you want to come with me?" I put my hands on each side of her face, forcing her to look at me. "Don't you love me anymore? I've missed you so!" Her tongue darted out, licking my hand. She wagged her tail and then struggled to get away from my hold on her.

Dad stood waiting, his intense blue eyes watching. No one said a word and the silence stretched on. I stood frozen, not knowing what to do.

Finally Dad said, "Well, Rachel, do we take her?"

"She doesn't want to come, Dad," I cried. "She doesn't want to come!"

Dad shut the door to the old sheep wagon and I sobbed in sorrow. I couldn't take Nisha if she didn't want to come. Maybe I couldn't have taken her from the old man anyhow. I knew now why Dad hadn't wanted to tell me he'd found her. Maybe I'd have been happier never knowing she preferred another person to me.

Once the sobs stopped, I leaned over and opened the door. "You can keep her, Mr. McIntosh," I said.

I shut the door without saying goodbye to Nisha. We walked back to our car in silence. Then Dad said, "Nisha still loves you,

Rachel, but now she knows old McIntosh needs her the most. Nisha's special and we were lucky to have had her for even a little while. And I'm so proud of you, Rachel, so very proud."

I hugged my warm coat around me against the cool breeze that seeped through the many cracks in the old car. The knot in my throat eased, but we were almost home before I spoke. "Do you think it's too late to make friends with Licorice?"

Sleet

by

Barbara Lau

Listen.
It is the litany
of motion stopping
the sizzle
of sky congealing
the slush
of curb against wheel

and the white hush
of my voice stalled
at the window like
a leaf clamped tight
in a closet of glass

the world at last
resolved
transfixed
like a branch bent with ice
like a nun bent in prayer.

Advice from My Uncle Tom

by

J. Jordan Cannady

When my Great-Uncle Tom Edward (the drinking uncle) found out I was to be married, he sent me the following message:

Jordan,

I've been a bachelor for nearly seventy years and consider myself an expert in the field of women. I don't want to meddle in your life but I feel I must warn you of one thing. No matter how slight your fault, miniscule your flaw, insignificant your mistake, your wife will feel morally bound to tell you what you've done wrong. Have a happy wedding. I won't be there.

Love,

Uncle Tom

I know he meant the best; still, I thought better about showing it to my bride-to-be. Maybe after the honeymoon, I thought. For how could I explain Tom to her? Uncle Tom had been sharing his opinions with the young men of the family for generations. One of my favorites was a tale about attending his first boy-girl dance.

198

Tom described the physical torture endured at the hands of his mother as he was plucked, preened, pruned, and spruced in anticipation of this gala event. His hair was slicked down with Brylcreme, his skin scrubbed raw with a soap made out of volcanic rock, his ears were invaded with the rough, twisted corner of a terry cloth washcloth and every nook, crevice, and cranny had been detailed. In short, Tommy felt like a deck of cards that had just been through a three-day magician's convention.

Tommy was dressed as if he were to be laid out in an adolescent funeral parlor. He wore a light blue and white striped seersucker suit, a white shirt with a collar stiff as a Methodist, a dark blue clip-on bow tie, and a tight pair of oxblood colored wing tips—the style you might see on the feet of a bookkeeper.

When done, he was thrust out of the bedroom into the waiting clutches of the gaggle of maiden aunts, sisters, mothers, grandmothers anxious to inspect him. He was passed along from one female to the next, struggling as his ears were peeled back, his hair tugged and spit-slicked, nails checked for dirt and biting, and the other endless flaws inherently found in boys. "I would have run if there hadn't been so many of them," Uncle Tom explained.

I thought of my Uncle Tom as I walked out to the car that would take me to my wedding. He'd be sitting in the corner of the hallway by the umbrella stand and hat rack, I figured. He'd reach out, grab me under the bow tie, and pull me through to him like a rag doll through a picket fence in order to give me some last-minute advice.

I still remember the rich masculine smell of him and his bourbon-soaked tobacco, wool suit, the emerald green tonic he used on his hair, and the spice of Bay Rum aftershave intermingled with three-year-old Kentucky sour mash. He'd pull me in close and look me straight in the eyes, man to man.

"Young man," he'd say, 'I'm going to tell you something about women that I don't want you to ever forget.' The way he'd say it, I would know that this was to be one of those few truly epiphanous moments in life where some mystery was to be made clear.

But what would he say? Then I heard him: "Always remember boy, when it comes to women, the dumbest one out there is smarter than you'll ever be."

With that and a sly, conspiratorial wink, he'd give me a gentle push back into the crowd. As I continued through the gauntlet, I'd look back toward my Uncle Tom. He'd stick his left arm out away from his side, fold his right arm across his chest, and give me a smile as he'd sway back and forth in his chair in a solitary dance. I'd see my bride-to-be and then I'd know why he'd backed down. I'd look back at him and he'd be tearing up that warning he'd been thinking of sending.

Nice Car

by

Kathleen Hoffman

It's a strange thing, and probably very much American, the hold cars can have on their owners.

Here they are, masses of steel and rubber and gauges and things that can disconnect, break, blow out, come apart, fall off, and so on, and people form these tremendous attachments to them. They wash, polish, and dote on their cars. Drivers who normally won't walk ten steps will park a half mile from a mall entrance to be sure no one opens a door into the shiny paint on their autos, and unmarried people who give rides to friends with children go into more of a snit when the kids drip stuff onto the upholstery than they would if someone broke the windows on their house.

Then, when it's time to get a new car, and go through the long-distance parking and protective behavior against three-year-olds again, these same people have a terrible time trading in their old friend. "Maybe it's got another year or two in it," they'll say, looking at ragged seats, rusted sides, and scraped doors.

I had such an old friend, only I didn't get it when it was new. It was in 1971 that my husband and I, married only a few years and facing the fact that I needed a car so I could return to work after the birth of our child, began looking for "cheap transporta-

201

tion." We found it, $300 cheap—a white Ford Falcon, a 1963 model, already with fairly high mileage.

We'd only have it a few years, we told ourselves, until we could afford something better. We held that thought when my husband drove it off the road on an icy curve the first winter we had it. Those dents didn't matter—the ones it got scraping along the ditch before it bounded out again—because we'd only have it for a few years.

But it turned out that in going off the road, the Falcon had already demonstrated its one drawback—it didn't drive well in really bad weather. Other than that it was a vehicular form of that old joke about the washing machine that the manufacturer found in an old lady's house, still working after forty years. "Pay her whatever you have to, but bring that washer into the research lab," he ordered. "Then go over it, inch by inch, bolt by bolt. I want to know what made it work for forty years." Once the puzzle was solved, he said, the company would have the most valuable knowledge it could come up with. "We'll never, never, make another one like it," he swore.

That's what that little white car was. It started with a hand choke, and once you got the hang of using it, the Falcon always started. I used to drive it on the job at a small-town newspaper, and in my comings and goings I would often crank it up a dozen times a day. In all the time we had it, it failed to start only twice—and on one of those occasions it had given a definite, throat-clearing warning that it was going to have trouble, that the battery was in dire need of replacement. It also chose a spot two blocks from a service station in which to get serious about the bad battery.

Its parts were solid and trustworthy. Once we were in a six-car chain reaction collision. Actually, I managed not to hit the car in front of me when it hit the one in front of it, but the van behind me slammed into the Falcon's back bumper. When the police looked over the damage, the van's bumper was bent in against its blunt snout, but the Falcon showed only a bit of blue paint from the van's front. The policeman grinned at me, and didn't even bother to add us to his report.

Actually, to say its snow aversion was its only fault is exagger-

202

ating a bit. As it grew older, it developed a few other quirks. It was an automatic, but you couldn't put it in park, because it would get stuck. Therefore I always looked for flat places to park it (the emergency brake was less than trustworthy). Often the driver's side door would only work if you turned the button to a particular point before pushing it in. And, it did eat tailpipes, wearing them out with alarming regularity.

It was a car that had seat belts added as an afterthought, and it came with an American flag decal in the back window, firmly attached with that old-fashioned stickiness that never came off, and rode so high above the ground that it could go easily over places where ordinary cars scraped the ground.

One day, a co-worker, leaning on her shiny forest-green Volvo, looked at me getting out of the Falcon in the newspaper's parking lot and remarked, very quietly, "Nice car." From then on, it was always spoken of that way. Nice Car continued to go to and from work after we moved farther into the country, and it continued to start, always. We attributed its trustworthiness, as the years went on, partly to the fact that it had to pass a large and unseemly auto junkyard on the way to our new house. The odometer broke at about 38,000 miles, the second time around, of course, and after that we never knew how many miles it piled up.

But sadly, Nice Car began to rust through its paint. We declined to have it painted, knowing it would not survive the procedure, act of faith that it would be. Finally, and suddenly, its motor developed a problem too bad for ordinary remedies. Just another tailpipe wasn't going to be enough this time.

The answer was a transplant. A motor from another Falcon was installed, this one so ill-used that its horn was honked with a button taped to the dashboard. It went on and on with a new lease on life that lasted several years.

Then the brakes went. They were fixed. Then they went again, allowing me to experience the unfortunate feeling of free fall in a car. They were fixed, but when they went out a third time, Nice Car took my husband across four lanes of traffic into a deep ravine on the other side—safely, thankfully, but he took it badly.

It was time. We picked out another car that on the inside

looked just about like Nice Car, and made arrangements to simply leave the Falcon at the dealer's. They snickered when someone used the term "trade-in." On that last day that we had the Falcon, we added brake fluid, and it started shakily. Loyally it made the trip to the dealership. I followed in the other car—in case it didn't manage to cover the eight miles—and watched its sturdy little upright self head up the road. It was very sad, regardless of the fact that I was about to start an equally fierce and unsuitable attachment to its replacement, a 1976 primer-gray Maverick that was one of the ugliest cars ever built.

A couple of months later, I watched as a boy in a Hardee's uniform got out of a small white Falcon at a mall fifty miles away. I surreptitiously checked it out—yep, rusty ditch-scraped fenders, sticky decal remains in the back window, a tailpipe about ready to fall off. No question, it was Nice Car!

I suppressed the impulse to mug the lad and reclaim my friend. For everything, there is a season, but the season of Nice Car was a vehicular highlight and we will never quite see its like again.

Green Symphony

by

Ingrid Reti

I sit sipping mint tea
the soft green leaves
picked last summer
and now
after the first rainstorm
looking at the freshly dressed green hills
I celebrate life
remembering
once long ago
climbing a fence
climbing a tree
relishing the tartness of a green apple;
grass stains on a party dress
mint frosting on a birthday cake
my mother's shiny rubber tree.

I sit sipping mint tea
remembering so many things;
that first Christmas in Venezuela

a single decorated evergreen branch
wilting in the tropical heat;
a shiny green iguana immobile
on our garden wall;
years later,
a hike through a forest of towering ferns
one Christmas in New Zealand.

I sit sipping mint tea
celebrating life
thinking of Lassen vistas;
the wind in my hair,
the swaying tall grasses on Mt. Harkness
the transient green of snow-melt lakes;
a baby fir tree rescued
from its stifling snow blanket;
our kelly green tent facing Lassen Peak
and I, in the midst of a green meadow
watching whitecaps race across Juniper Lake.

I sit sipping mint tea
remembering so many things.
the Vietnam War and the Green Berets;
my garden scissors terminating
a green tomato caterpillar;
tiny pet green turtles dying,
explaining death to a child.

I sit celebrating life.

Peaches

by

Allan George Whitfield

It was 1946 and Brooklyn in August was as boring to me as one of
Reverend Melish's sermons. Most of the guys were away at camp
or vacationing with their parents. Louie was the only other regular from our gang who was home. There hadn't been a stickball
game in three weeks. We didn't even play *Ring-a-leave-e-o* after supper, just sat around, drank Mission Orange, and told lies.

One afternoon, Louie and I were on the prowl. For prowl-
ing, Fifth Avenue was the place to be. That was where the action
was. Bars, shops, trolleys.

Trolleys ran down the center of the Avenue, two sets of
tracks, one going to South Brooklyn, the other out to Fort Hamil-
ton where the Army base was. We'd wait until trolleys approached
from opposite directions and at the last instant, dash between
them. The motormen would clang their bells and shake their fists
at us. It was *great!*

There were two bars between 46th and 47th Streets, Duffy's
and Johnson's. They faced each other across the Avenue, neon
lights winking seductively. A drunk, ejected from one joint, could
try his luck in the other.

The shops were our targets as we shuffled along. We
touched everything that was on sidewalk display. Sometimes the

touch became a grasp and we "treated" ourselves to something just for the thrill of stealing it.

Tony's vegetable store was a good place to do some real touching. Apples, peaches, and kumquats were easily grabbed and didn't slow us down if we were spotted and had to make a run for it.

This day on the sidewalk, Tony had bushel baskets filled with ripe peaches. As we drew closer, an idea took shape in my eleven-year-old mind: we should relieve Tony of a whole bushel of peaches. My scalp tightened and tingled with excitement.

I grabbed Louie's arm and steered him across the street. "I've gotta great idea. The peaches, let's take a whole basket."

"You're nuts, Al! Those things must weigh a hundred pounds," Louie said.

"You're chicken, Lou," I taunted. "I'll do it myself!"

"You can't," he protested. "You'll never get it off the ground."

After five minutes of fierce argument, Louie agreed to be the second hand on the basket handles. The strategy was set: make sure Tony was in the back of the store, grab the handles, run down Fifth Avenue to 46th Street, up 46th to Sixth Avenue, down Sixth Avenue to the park—home free!

We waited across the street where we could see Tony. I was keyed up, anxious to get on with it.

After what seemed like hours, Tony followed a customer to the back of his store. This was our chance. "*Now,* Lou!"

We darted across the street and swooped down on a bushel basket, grabbed the handles, and yanked. The thin wire handles cut into our hands.

"Move it," I gasped.

We tightened our grips and began to run. My heartbeat quickened with the first stride and escalated to a war-dance once our four feet were in motion, the basket swaying between us.

I was a good five inches taller than Louie. The difference in height caused the basket to tilt, making our burden seem heavier than it was. However, the power of evil and fear of Italian retribution pushed our adrenalin to the limit as we ran down Fifth Avenue to-ward 46th Street, peaches spilling onto the sidewalk behind us.

A drunk staggered out of Johnson's Bar and began throwing up in front of us. Like a well-oiled machine, we reacted as one, veering smartly into the street to avoid the mess. Once past it we bounced back onto the sidewalk and continued on.

Turning the corner on 46th, we headed toward Sixth Avenue. I felt powerful, as though I could do anything, vanquish any foe, win any battle, steal any fruit.

Louie, who was never my first choice in stickball, was actually holding up his side of the basket very well. As we neared Sixth Avenue, I wanted to give up, but, thank God for pride, I wouldn't quit before Louie did.

Just when I felt we couldn't run another step, we were inside cool, green Sunset Park. I led the way to my favorite hiding place, a huge bush which, once inside, completely hid us from notice.

Our hands burned from the deep red grooves in our palms; we couldn't drop the basket fast enough. We flung ourselves on the ground, gasping for breath. I thought my sides would burst.

After a while breathing slowed and the pain lessened.

"Do you think anyone saw us, Al?" Louie asked.

"Nah," I said, not entirely sure I was right.

"We did it!" Louie shouted.

We felt triumphant and giddy as the magnitude of what we had done sank in. One self-congratulatory phrase after another escaped our lips:

"Great, we're great!"

"Did you see the drunk's face when we whizzed by!"

"Was that a great idea, or what!"

"If we were in the war, we could have stole Hitler!"

"To the victor belong the spoils!"

I bit into the first peach. It was everything I could have hoped for—sweet, juicy...stolen.

Many peaches later, Louie whined, "I've gotta get home, Al."

"Me, too," I said, knowing it would soon be suppertime, but not wanting to eat again, ever.

We crawled out of our green fort, leaving behind the basket and the few remaining peaches. My stomach was bloated and my head ached. "I'll never eat another peach as long as I live," I vowed.

"Me, neither," Louie whimpered.

When we parted, there were no winks, slaps on the back, or other expressions of a great adventure shared. Just two sick and sorry boys heading for bathrooms.

"What have you been up to, Pal?" Grampa asked as I came in the front door.

"Nothin', Pop. I don't feel so good; can I go to bed?" I headed for the bathroom.

Twenty minutes later, somewhat relieved, I walked into the kitchen where Gramma performed the inevitable physical examination.

She had come to America from Norway, still had a heavy Norwegian accent, and couldn't understand American slang and idioms. She believed that Castoria, a laxative, would cure most ailments.

She took my temperature, felt my head, and held my wrist for a moment. Then she looked at Grampa and pronounced me, "Sick vit an oopset stoomick! Get the Castoria!"

I dragged myself up the stairs to my bedroom, an act I would repeat many times that night. It seemed like an endless process— bathroom, bed, bathroom, bed. Finally to sleep. My nightmares were of baskets, bushes, and bathrooms. When I awoke, that queasy feeling—peach excess—was still with me.

I entered the kitchen, sat at the table and greeted my Grandmother weakly, "Morning, Gramma."

"Good morning. You poor thing. Since you ver so sick last night and couldn't eat, I have a treat for your breakfast. Your favorite. Corn flakes vit peaches."

The Cry of the Jay

by

M.A. Schaffner

The real spring snuck in again this year, surprising everyone and making Elliot feel, as he does every year, just a little foolish at being surprised. Sure, the bats had already been out for a while, and he and Martha had had that great day in the park some weeks back, but then the cold returned, and after two or three more hot days, there had been another freeze.

April Fools' Day had already slipped by. All Fools' Day. Even the name fits the season well. Cold Canadian winds and Bermuda-bred thunderstorms alternate with the distracting speed of cards in a sharper's deck. When the first real spring day hits, it's a bit like sitting on that whoopie cushion you know you would've spotted if you hadn't just been talking to the guy with the stupid smile who'd put it there.

Every year this happens, and almost just this way. Every year Elliot would go through the same period of trading topcoat for trench coat for sport coat alone. He'd wonder whether winter would come back or if we'd jump straight into the hell of a humid July, and he'd never guess till the last that, yes boys and girls, we *will* have a spring. Crocuses are tentative, daffodils are just signs; it takes the day that everything explodes for you to really know.

And now, one early evening just past six, as Elliot walked home down Zachary Street, he knew the day had come. In one day the hyacinths had jumped out, the forsythia had caught fire, a delicate fringe of bright green had edged the outstretched branches of old trees, and the good citizens of Arlington County had lined the streets with bags of lawn debris. And he remembered that early that morning a flicker had come back to a house three blocks down to hammer its jackhammer song on the rain gutter.

Elliot walked down the street and listened to the other new sounds. An old couple sat on a porch swing and argued as expertly as only two people who've lived together for half a century can. Young mothers chatted over their baby carriages. A neighbor's girl stood in the middle of the street by her boyfriend's car, her conversation with him hidden behind a wall of deep car-radio rhythms. A block from the house, a horde of grackles filled the boughs of three neighboring oaks with the thin screams of rusty hinges. Next door, the old cat crept out from under the bushes and brushed Elliot's legs in a sly demand for tribute. Elliot complied with a pet and the cat purred. Later, at home, after Elliot got changed and went out back with a drink to see what Martha had to show him in the garden, he was greeted by a trio of blue jays calling out from the mulberry.

Martha stopped and looked where Elliot looked, both of them searching as if their eyes could up the volume or bring the birds closer for a better view. The three jays strutted, bold and electric blue, dashing ambassadors of the strange bright world that hides in the open all around us.

Elliot watched one jay as it cocked its head and underscored a question with its long black beak. It moved a foot for a steadier stance then reared back and cried again, a piercing metallic shout evocative of some special jay emotion that springs from murky sources somewhere between alarm and triumph, innocence and guile. The jay looked down, noticed Elliot, and cocked its head again. *Neither of us*, Elliot thought, *has the faintest idea what it's like to be the other, though we might meet again and again throughout the warm months. But it won't matter. I'll go back to the office and know*

212

that this is one area of ignorance that I need never account for. And the jay won't even be able to pose the question. But on the other hand, it can fly.

"I wonder what he's saying," Martha mused.

"It's spring. One of the other two is probably a female. You figure it," Elliot replied helpfully.

"Maybe that's why she's not answering," Martha said.

He muttered and they returned to the garden tour. All the while Elliot listened to the birds singing solos over Martha's continuo, and looked from his garden, with its japonica and nandina to cardinal and house finch as the latter darted from branch to feeder and porch rail to fence.

There was something intriguing in the struggle of new plants rising from the mulch and unfolding in the sun, but there was something even more compelling in the appearance of the birds. Birds vacation in sunny places all winter and then bring some of that sun back with them. Their songs are tales of long sunsets in South Florida and the Caribbean. Where had Elliot gone that winter? Downtown, to cold asphalt and sparse clumps of green that curled upon themselves trying to get away from traffic. *That's what you get for an opposable thumb,* he thought, looking at a cardinal. It laughed.

It wasn't easy to work the next day. He had a window office and could see a little patch of park nearby. Some sadists from the Park Service had put tulips out to torment all the office workers. At lunch Elliot went to a Thai restaurant with a supervisor he thought he should get to know better. He ended up spending seven dollars on sautéed watercress and an hour inside, when the whole time he could have been sitting in that park for free, listening to the bums talk politics and watching the tulips grow.

For a passing moment on the walk back, he thought of asking his supervisor if he wouldn't mind getting a bottle of wine and having a little staff meeting under the magnolia next to the bronze hero; but the supervisor was talking about the Performance Management Recognition System and the moment was suddenly gone. When they got back, the supervisor needed to

213

have a response to a department written, and he dumped it on Elliot.

Elliot spent the rest of the afternoon pulling files, fabricating authoritative statements, cursing the boss, and watching Park Service gardeners in deep green uniforms taunt him from the light green grass a block away.

He was in a foul mood coming home. He imagined the old people on their porch escalating their argument with assault rifles and sending a few stray rounds into the yuppie mothers with the baby carriages. The thought made him smile. He imagined the grackles caught in a cloud of Iraqi mustard gas and their rusty hinged cries ebbing into barely audible squeaks. Hee hee.

On the flicker's hill, two kids, maybe five years old, were making a game of tossing old spiky sweet gum pods at each other and passersby. It was a harmless game and their delight was evident as they watched Elliot's approach and shared innocent conspiratorial giggles. He fingered the Swiss army knife in his pocket and muttered, "Mess with me and I'll cut your wicked little hearts out, you pint-sized savages." They didn't hear, but they saw. They fled into the next yard like fairies at sunrise.

But it was Friday. Elliot got home and poured a drink and sat out on the porch to listen to Martha and watch the jays. The three jays danced and sang through the mulberry and the neighboring trees. Down below, the old cat watched, licked its paw, then stalked away.

Odd thing about jays, Elliot thought. They're so big and bold, but when the warm days come on and the cat gets about, you'll as soon find the cat with one of the jays as with a sparrow. You wouldn't think so. There were a lot more sparrows and they didn't seem particularly bright. They had a habit, for example, of building nests in the stovepipe. All spring and during parts of other seasons, Elliot would have to fetch them out when they fell down into the firebox. Every year they made at least one complete nest that ended up falling down the pipe. One fall, as Elliot went to play chimney-sweep, he found a half dozen fully or partially constructed nests scrunched together at the bottom with their occupants. He stopped counting bodies at fifteen. Martha

214

never let him forget it. Every time a visitor oohed or aahed over the quaint wood stove, she casually referred to it as "Dr. Elliot's Chamber of Death." It got on his nerves.

But the point of it all was that sparrows were not half the birds jays seemed to be. So how come, whenever he weeded the beds or spread the mulch, Elliot was as likely to come across the broken-necked form of an electric-blue prince as the black-bibbed corpse of a commoner? One of nature's mysteries, no doubt. He could go to his encyclopedia and trace the kings of the Capetian dynasty, or the latest atomic theories at the time of publication, but that little secret would remain. Right now he dismissed it with another drink, leaned back, and listened to the songs.

"How long do you think we'll have three of them?" Martha asked. Elliot was a little surprised. He didn't realize she'd been watching them too.

"I don't know," he replied. "I don't suppose jays go in for threesomes."

"We'll see," she said.

"Yeah, maybe we can learn something," he continued.

"I doubt it," Martha finished.

Saturday was warm and fine. A good day for weeding and turning over soil. Funny how fascinating dirt can be after you spend a week in an office. Earlier in the week, Elliot joked to co-workers about the joy of gardening. He said things like how much fun it was to be mindless for a change, to dig in dirt instead of paper. But he had come to realize that that was something of a lie. It was really the office work that had become mindless. He was now at that level of expertise or boredom at which he could handle nearly any problem placed on his desk on autopilot, the recitation of advice and regulatory citations flowing from his lips like the words of the mass from an eighty-year-old priest's.

Dirt, on the other hand, involved a whole new set of un-guessed skills. Just turning over soil presented choices. You could use a long-handled shovel, a gardener's spade, or a cultivator. You could break up the clods with heavy tines or the edge of a blade. Tools could be swung or dropped or pushed or pulled. The reas-surance that this was work, real work, came stronger and deeper from the feel of hands on oiled wood, not from fingertips on plastic keys. Also, weeds were challenges requiring different approaches according to the soil and how they managed to grip it. A little maple seedling in a well-turned bed would come up with the lightest pull; a wild strawberry in packed clay demanded a good grip on the base of the stem and a steady pull with strong fingers. Elliot used a metal weeder on plantains and dandelions, getting as much of the roots as he could, but not worrying about what might be left behind. Sure, a dandelion would come back from a tiny bit of root, but only so often, and Elliot planned to be there each time.

He knelt in the pathway of the vegetable plot, deep in the soil and deeper in his thoughts of dirt and weeds. He wrote a little treatise in his mind and addressed an imaginary crowd of colleagues on the delicate tasks of the gardener as he plucked at seedlings and smelled the life emanating from the blooming earth. Then, as he brushed a layer of last fall's leaves from a patch of ground ivy, he confronted what at first seemed to be a big earthworm. Very soon he saw that it was too big, and as it coiled into a writhing heap, he recognized it as a garter snake. *Hello*, he thought, as he grabbed it just behind the head and carried it to the compost heap. With a nod to a garden long since shut down, he thought, *How nice to meet a serpent that keeps its mouth shut.*

Elliot let the snake go and watched it sink into the steaming mound of clippings and table scraps. He was starting another lecture in his mind, this time on the topic of helpful and unhelpful serpents, when he was startled by a thump on the turf behind him. It sounded like a kid had thrown an old tennis ball that fell short of its mark. He turned around, half-alarmed and ready to lecture aloud. But there on the grass a blue jay lay on its side, one wing oddly twisted. It looked a little surprised.

Elliot had no idea what to do. He looked up, as if there might be an answer there. Maybe the jay had fallen out of a tree. But there weren't any branches overhead. It must have just fallen out of the sky. No. Could it? He looked down again. The jay shook itself and got up on its feet. Obviously it couldn't fly.

The thing to do, Elliot thought, was get a shoe box, put it in,

216

and keep it until it got better. He was about to call Martha, thinking, how will this sound? *Martha, Martha, quick, get a shoe box!*

Then the jay presented him with a new dilemma by hopping off behind an azalea. Damn. You can't let it go. What about the cat? Eliot walked up to the bird, slow and quiet, wondering if his gloves were up to the challenge of the beak of a frightened jay. The jay turned its head, clacked that big black beak, and squeaked a squawk that sounded like fingers on a blackboard. Elliot shivered, took another step, and it bounded off around the house to the front yard. *Come on, I'm trying to help*, Elliot thought as he followed the bird. He wondered how he must look, half bent over and pursuing a hopping bird as quickly and stealthily as he could in gardening clogs. It crossed the neighbor's driveway. Elliot stayed with it, still bent over, till the neighbor's voice arrested him. The neighbor had been watching from his front porch.

"Hey there, Elliot," he said, "what're you after?"

"Ah, a blue jay," Elliot answered. "Fell down in the yard and hurt its wing. I'm trying to find it." He caught a glimpse of blue in the shadows of the next house's shrubs. It vanished.

"Probably fighting," the neighbor said, shaking his head. "They do that this time of year, you know. You won't find him, Elliot. Not unless the cat brings him home for you."

Elliot looked once more at the spot where he last saw the jay. He knew Fred was right and that the next time he saw the jay it would be just like the others: stiff-necked and faded in a patch of old leaves. And soon after that he would see the old cat and it would lick its paws, curl his legs, and then go back to its bowl for milk. Then the leaves would fall and it would be cold and gray until the next day the earth decided to explode into many colors. And on that day he would be surprised again.

Somewhere in the shadows before him a pair of dark eyes glanced furtively at the light and something small and princely shuddered. But from above and behind, in the depths of the newly budded mulberry limbs, came a harsh metallic cry, a call of guileless triumph.

Memories of Finch Field

by

Don Gardner

Dad and I were on our way to Finch Field to see a doublehitter. I
didn't know much about baseball in the beginning and asked
how two hitters could bat at the same time. "Double *header*, son,"
my dad corrected. "That means two games, not two hitters."

Dad and I attended all the games at Finch Field to see our
beloved Hi-Toms play baseball. I could hardly wait for him to
come home. Dad was rushed through many meals while I impatiently waited, sighing pointedly if he poured a second glass of
iced tea. I liked to get there early to watch infield and batting
practice.

In 1948 the Hi-Toms had great pitching and power hitting.
"Junior" Leonard and Guy Prater were my heroes. Leonard had a
beautiful swing; when he hit a long, high-arcing fly ball, Dad and
I would jump to our feet and wait breathlessly while the out-
fielder raced to the fence and leapt at the last moment with outstretched glove as the baseball disappeared over the fence,
tantalizingly out of reach.

Prater was a terror to pitchers. He seemed six feet wide
through his shoulders and his arms bulged with muscles. When
he connected on a pitch, we knew instantly the ball was going for
a long ride. My brother Bobby saw a game where he claimed

218

Prater hit a ball over the light pole in right field...but Bobby probably stretched that story a little.

We had fun with our bat boy, Egolly. Whenever he went on the field to deliver baseballs to the umpire, Dad and I would shout in unison, "By golly, there's Egolly!"

And on the nights when our pitcher was sharp, the best fun was the goose—a large, white mechanical gander that slowly waddled its way across the scoreboard, squawking insolently over the P.A. system as it dramatically laid an egg when the visiting team failed to score.

In the middle of the third inning, Dad would buy soft drinks and a bag of roasted peanuts. I liked to shell the peanuts and put them in my drink—skins on or off, it didn't matter. After taking a swallow, there were always a few peanuts to chew on. On payday nights, Dad would treat me to a box of Cracker Jacks. At the bottom of the box was a prize I would inevitably lose the next day.

Baseball consumed me during all of my waking hours when I was a young boy. My favorite game was to hit rocks in our driveway, pretending I was winning crucial games for the Hi-Toms. My left-field wall was a fence at the back of our lot, extending into straightaway center field. In the middle of right field was a neighbor's house, which somewhat messed up my Finch Field, so I concentrated on hitting to left. Being a right-handed batter, that's where my power was anyway.

Each imaginary game ended with me rounding the bases after hitting the winning home run, always remembering to tip my hat modestly to the cheering fans, especially to the pretty girls who sat near our dugout.

When I grew up and married, I brought my wife to see the Hi-Toms. The home plate umpire had a rip—a major league rip—in the seat of his pants; when he leaned forward to call the next pitch, he flashed a magnificent view of white underwear. Between laughter we tried to call this to his attention, but several entertaining innings passed before the umpire understood what we were yelling to him.

As an adult, I visited a few major league stadiums, always pleased by the sights, sounds, and aura of a baseball park. I saw

Ted Williams and Fenway's wall in Boston. Ted's swing reminded me of Junior Leonard. I watched the Philadelphia Athletics play one long-ago weekend. Several decades later, with my sons Rick and Mark, we watched as the owner of the twice-removed Athletics presented Vida Blue with a new car the day after he pitched a no-hitter.

My sons and I were in D.C. Stadium one night when Frank Howard hit a home run deep into the center field seats. Whenever "Hondo" hit one of those giant home runs, a seat was painted white the next day to show where the ball had landed.

Mark and I were in Memorial Stadium the afternoon Brooks Robinson retired from playing baseball. My boys and I attended a few games at Dodger Stadium, and we also saw the minor league San Jose Bees play (their clubhouse was named the "Beehive").

At the beginning of the present baseball season, I decided to re-visit Finch Field. I knew that a professional baseball team had not played there for many years, but I wasn't prepared for the sight that awaited me.

Decay was everywhere. Numerous dingy industrial shops occupied what had once been the parking lot. Entire sections of outfield fence had either fallen or were hanging on by a few rusty nails; weeds covered the playing field. The tall light poles seemed to stand as forlorn beacons, waiting to be illuminated again for a night game. Peeling sheets of old gray paint hung loosely from the wooden grandstand, which seemed to creak and groan, as if ready to give up the ghost.

1948 was the season I remember best, but it ended tragically. The Hi-Toms were in first place and playing well when Leonard and Prater were banned from organized baseball (the newspaper didn't provide specifics). We finished in fourth place.

After all these years—decades, really—I still cannot bear to think of that event. Instead, I choose to recall the good times at Finch Field, remembering how I ran up the steps of the grandstand ahead of Dad, anxious to see the players on the field. I could almost hear the sounds of balls smacking into gloves, and the sharp crack of a bat followed by the sudden roar from the

220

fans. And there, behind the home dugout, is where the pretty girls sat to get a closer look at the handsome Eddie Matthews.

My plan was to walk onto the field and stride up to the plate as if I were batting. As a kid sitting in the stands, the outfield fence seemed to be a mile away. How much closer would it appear standing at home plate? Before stepping into the box, I thought to stand there for a moment and imagine how it might have been....

The gate was open, but I couldn't move. My feet seemed frozen in place, unable to carry me onto the field. Suddenly I felt embarrassed. Finch Field had once been a warm, special place for me, but now I felt I was standing on the grave of a loved one.

I drove quickly away, pursued by ghosts of bittersweet memories.

My Last Roundup

by

Nancy Climer

Our three-acre spread is sandwiched between a well-traveled, two-lane highway and a hundred or so fenced acres where a small herd of steers roam. Yesterday—a Sunday—I looked outside and saw one of those steers looking wistfully at his fellows. He was outside the electric wire fence that is intended to keep him in and quite outside our fence as well. I yelled the news of this to my husband, then phoned the farmer whose cattle these are, and high-tailed it outside.

The steer stood right beside the gate, which was a stretch of electrically charged wire with a mitt-sized black plastic handle. The handle was there to protect the person maneuvering said wire from shock (a stronger person than I, I discovered, for I couldn't get enough muscle on the thing to pull it out of the loop that served as its latch).

But it didn't matter now. The steer had decided to move down our fence line toward the highway. My husband ran down the drive and managed to get to the road. I circled wide as fast as I could and joined him there. The steer kept coming, even as, behind us, traffic whizzed by in both directions.

The steer began to trot. He was bent on dodging past us. I could see this intention in his eye and in the way he shifted as we did, a little to the right, a little to the left. My husband and I, with some inborn Texas instinct neither of us knew we possessed, began hooting and gesturing. At what seemed the last possible instant, the steer swerved, and all we had to do was hold our position until the farmer arrived.

But where was he? We asked this more and more heatedly, until at last the man's dusty white pickup rolled into view. He and his wife tumbled out, so disheveled that we knew they'd been sleeping in on this particular morning. Rope in hand, they advanced on the steer.

But then the farmer called to his wife and the two spoke softly before turning back to the spot where we stood. "This steer," the farmer said, "he's not one of mine."

I began to sputter and I assumed the additional sputtering that I heard came from my husband. "Mine," the farmer went on, "have their ears notched and this one doesn't. Mine…"

"I believe you," I interrupted him. "But we can't just leave this animal wandering around." The farmer and his wife agreed. They rousted the steer through a little side gate into our front yard. "What now?" I wanted to know. The farmer muttered something about checking with someone or other and he and his wife drove off.

Hours later the steer was still in our front yard, alternately mooing and braying, the latter a sound I hadn't known steers could make. I offered it water and watched as it overturned the bucket and rattled it hither and yon. Better the bucket, I thought, than the parsley and chives and basil I had planted.

Meanwhile, our son telephoned to say he'd be in the neighborhood and would stop by. "There's a steer in the front yard," I told him, relishing, at least, the prospect of recounting the tale. "So," I said, struggling to maintain a matter-of-fact tone, "be careful when you come in through the gate."

Our son said one word, a flat "Okay."

It was equally anticlimactic but nonetheless a relief when, about four hours later, a red and white king cab truck drove up and several men emerged from it. One of them tipped his gimme cap and uttered a "Thank you ma'am" in my direction. The others blocked traffic on the highway while the steer was headed out that way, presumably toward its rightful home.

My husband and son? They were inside, watching a cowboy movie on TV.

Cora

by

Sally Bellerose

Grandmother Cora said that each person gets allotted so many foolish words at birth and after they're all used up the person dies. Nana, as we called her, lived next door, alone, in the house where she had raised five sons and one daughter. Mama let me spend most of my time in Nana's old house. Mama had a new baby and my older brother and sister to take care of at home.

Nana had married at sixteen and lived with Papa Pepe until he passed away, sixty years later. When Papa Pepe died, I was very young, four or five. I remember him yelling my grandmother's name, "Cora, I'm cold," and Nana would cover him with the muslin quilt she was forever mending. He was bedridden at the end.

Nana tried to warn him, "You'll kill yourself with all that racket."

He persisted, focusing every want and need in her name.

"Cora!" We could hear him yell as we jumped rope in the next yard.

I sang and danced at his funeral. Nana clapped her hands to break up the sorrow. We sang,

> Jimmy Crack Corn and I don't care
> Jimmy Crack Corn and I don't care

Jimmy Crack Corn and I don't care
My master's gone away

Then long hours of silence with Nana all to myself.

If I spoke too much, she would say gently, but in French, "Shut your mouth." From Nana it was a soothing remark. After saying it, she would always kiss my mouth. She would rock, humming prayers on her rosary beads. I rarely spoke; I sang. In Nana's house you could sing anything, anything sad, or funny, or foolish, as long as you didn't sing too loud. My favorites were her French songs. Memorized phrases, syllables strung together with no need for specific meaning. I sang. Nana rocked.

Some nights I slept with Nana in her big feather bed. The bed Papa Pepe had lived in. The bed he died in. Every morning Nana would sweep up a dustpan full of feathers. I took care not to bounce too hard on Nana's bed.

On weekends we played Nurse. Nana gave me a box of band-aids all my own. I cried when they were all used up. Then Nana cut *The Daily News* into little rectangles and stuffed them into the empty tin band-aid box. She tore up an old slip for more serious injuries. Nana was a good patient. She would lie still, to be nursed with tap-water potion from an old Coke bottle. Once Mama walked in while Nana was dying. Mama called me an unnatural child. Nana laughed. She knew I would always revive her.

Nana's eyesight was starting to go. She burned things, food, and her hands. Mama let me eat supper with her almost every night, just Nana and I. After supper Mama would ask, "What did you eat?" Nana would smile and I would make something up. Something with a vegetable in it. Really, we ate English muffins.

Nana would say, "I want blueberry pie tonight," and I would spread the thick blue jam on the muffins. She would say, "Shall we have a soufflé? I feel like a holiday," and I would fry two hamburgers to stack between the muffins.

One night Nana didn't want supper. She hadn't hummed *Alouette* for days.

"Come. Rock," she said. I was as tall as Nana by then. She

was much wider. I didn't see how I could sit on her without sliding off, so I sat on the floor and put my head in her lap.

"I'm ready to die," she said.

"I know, Nana." I did know. I knew Nana would be gone before I got old. I had been trying not to grow too fast.

"It's not so bad," she said. "You don't have to cry when the others do."

She left me then and began talking to all her dead relatives, foolish talk, to her husband, sisters, friends, her mama and papa, her own nana. On and on, sing-song, rocking.

She had used up all her words.

The Law of Women

by

Erik Bundy

I was almost sixteen years old when I started to teach in a sod-walled, one-room hut out on the windy Kansas prairie. That was about fifty years ago, just before the Civil War. Other than a teaching permit, all I owned of note was a black valise with three calico frocks, two slat bonnets, some womanly things, a fountain pen for writing poetry, a few sheets of fancy paper, a locket from my grandmother, and a clean Colt Navy .36 caliber pistol to scare off marauders.

On the first day of school, my heart fluttered like a bed sheet drying in the wind, especially when I clanged the clapper bell, shaking it with my whole right arm, to let the pupils know it was time to come in from the yard. I then stood at the front of the room with my head up to give a good appearance and was surprised at their reaction: they milled about just inside the door, staying clear of me, like I had smallpox or something. We all knew each other, of course, though I lived a ways off, and most of us had schooled together or played together at fairs and church socials, but now my place had changed. I was *the teacher*. Their shyness made me stiffen my spine even a bit more.

"All right, everybody sit," I ordered, "and we'll see what

books we've got." Since the school provided no texts, the learners brought what they could, mostly smudge-paged Bibles.

Everybody clunked a lard pail (with a lunch in it) down on the split log benches lining the two sidewalls of the schoolroom and sat—except for pig-headed Herman. I had known and not liked him for three years. He stood beside our fuel, which was a stack of cow chips—a fitting place for him.

"You deaf, Herman?" I asked.

He grinned. "You going to make me sit, Katie Ann?"

Vania Janssen dug at the hard dirt floor with a big toe. Nine Cheshire-cat grins, counting Herman's, mocked me. Most of the learners I could scrap with and win, but not with Herman Trefmann. He was only a year or two younger than I was and was strong enough to throw over a heifer. Besides which, the seams of my hand-me-down, butter-colored frock would rip if even frowned at strongly. And wrestling with a fool like Herman would put a hole in my discipline bigger than a doorway.

"Either that or kill you," I answered. I jerked the Colt Navy pistol out of my valise, cocked it, and aimed. He stood pillar-still, not believing I'd shoot. I could have parted his wispy blonde hair for him, but instead put a bullet into the soft wall about a foot above his shiny forehead. The noise nearly knocked the Van Witter twins off their log.

Herman hit the dirt floor like a dropped sack of feed. "You c-c-could a killed me!"

Smoke shaded the room. I examined my revolver, pretending I had made a bad shot. "Pisswilliker! I don't *usually* miss shots this close."

That bleached Herman's meaty face, even though he must have known I was an expert shot. Everybody in the county had heard my pa brag about my shooting. Still, being a target does scare a body beyond careful thinking.

Nobody smiled now.

And I didn't have a speck more trouble that week, even when I whipped the Adams boy for inking Vania's ponytail. He took his licking as easy as an old horse takes its harness. You should have seen the grateful look on his face when I reached for the caning rod instead of my six-shooter.

One boy who might have troubled me if given a chance was Ernest Redding. He had no ma, just an aunt who was kind to him only when she let him be, and a pa who didn't spare the rod. Ernest was immune to beatings, so I used my other weapon when I caught him de-trousering the Hawkins boy: I told him privately that if I caught him in any more mischief, I'd kiss him publicly. He turned red. A kiss, used at the right time (wrong time for people like him), can be just as powerful as a bullet.

The school term churned along like butter in the making—with a lot of ups and downs. Since the crops were already in the ground, most of the learners came every day. Each week I would stay at a different student's house; and two weeks, of course, with the Van Witter twins, there being two of them. My home was in the area, but was just too far a walk to make every day. Board was most of my pay, anyway.

After eight weeks came the Monday I dreaded. I had to board at Herman Trefmann's house..

The Trefmanns were thundering abolitionists, while most everyone else around Leavenworth, Kansas, held pro-slavery views. Herman's pa stuck out like a raisin in sourdough. The only reason I took Herman into my school was that his pa agreed to pay a dollar per month, which was double the usual rate. But part of the bargain had me boarding with them as if they were ordinary folk.

So that Monday, right after I let out school, Herman and I set off on the four-mile hike to the Trefmann homestead. I carried my own valise. For two miles we listened to the wind hiss. Around us stretched the storm-swept waste wrought from brown grass. Not a solitary tree or boulder relieved the eye. Over us hung an abandoned sky. The desolate prairie had a twin in Herman's empty head.

He muttered something.

"Speak up, if you've got something worth saying," I told him. "Only hogs ought to grunt."

"Don't see why we got to take in a slaver, is all," he said.

"It's the way things are done. Even my pa didn't kick up any

230

dust over my staying with you all. Any other time he'd boil me for fat."

Herman snorted, "They ain't a mite a fat on *your* bones. You're as skinny as a hoe handle and about near as plain. And you got cow-pie eyes. Just shows what you're stuffed with."

Herman was getting downright poetical.

"Leastwise," I said, "I don't smell musty like dung, which is more than can be said for you. And I'm thin, not skinny. I only just got my growth. Not everybody gets as much at the trough as you do, Herman Trefmann."

"You ain't even pretty," he shouted into the wind. "I could plow a field with your nose."

I shrugged. Why argue with a fool? "Being pretty out here just gets you babies quicker."

"You won't have none. What man wants a hoe handle?" he asked in a pig-mean tone. "That's why you teach school, ain't it? 'Cause no man has asked you to be his bride?"

I could have named two men who were interested. Trouble was, neither of them interested me. So I had set up a school. There was no other way for a woman of my talents to earn a living.

Herman's mother, Irmgard Trefmann waited out in a field for us. She was a broad German woman who twisted her hair up into a bun and refused to wear a bonnet. Her face reminded me of tree bark.

"What's wrong, Ma?" asked Herman. None of the other parents had walked out to greet me.

She nodded to me. "Welcome." Then she explained to Herman in broken English, "A gang of murderers look for your father, and he go to Topeka, and say, now you will hide here. So."

"Hide from slavers?" Herman grimaced like he had a bellyache.

I caught myself smiling. He hadn't thought himself so everlasting when my Colt threatened his mortality.

His ma looked at him with sorrow before saying in a skillet-hard voice, "You do like I tell you."

Herman didn't like being ordered about and looked as if he

wanted a mule to whip, but didn't have one nearby, so he motioned at me. "We going to keep her?"

"Mr. Trefmann give his word." Irmgard sighed. "*Mein Gott. Men kill over ideas. Is it not enough that wilderness kill us all?*"

The Trefmanns lived better than most, having an actual cabin with a porch for shade. They also owned a brimful well. Off to one side of their dusty yard huddled the sod hut they had lived in before their cabin was built. I was to stay there. A place all to myself was a luxury almost beyond belief.

Their cabin was one room, of course, with a plank floor and a cook stove standing solid in one corner. An oak table held the room's center while brass beds covered by comforters filled all three other corners.

Irmgard Trefmann laid out supper silently. She dismissed any need for my help. Herman's little brother and sister stared at me the whole while as if they had heard I danced naked under full moons. So it was a quiet meal, if you didn't count Herman's slurping. What was there to say? It was a time when many wives had to bury their husbands and move back East. Mr. Trefmann might be shot dead already. But the food was a joy. Irmgard Trefmann always won blue ribbons for her cooking at the county fairs. She could have boiled rocks and made them tasty.

I had figured she would hate me for her pain, but she seemed happy to entertain another woman. We did the washing up together. She even showed me what herbs made her soup so savory. And as I went out to the sod hut for the night, she patted my back and said, "You not to blame."

For a woman out on the windy prairie, loneliness carried the thorniest burden.

She made Herman carry my valise. "This is my place when you ain't in it," he muttered. It contained a brass bed and a small fireplace.

"You'll have it back in a week," I said.

"If I'm still alive then," he said. "Those rattlesnakes better not get Pa. I'll kill every one of them." His broad face flushed the red-brown color of old leather.

"Why'd your kind settle here in the first place?" I asked. "You knew this was a pro-slavery area."

"'Cause we can settle where we please," he answered.

"You ain't got the sense of a prairie dog," I said.

"Well, leastways," he asserted, "my kind don't treat others like pack mules."

"Sure you do. I've seen how your pa treats your ma. She ain't nothing more than a servant to him," I said.

I must have cut his pride, and he must have been more wrought up than I had imagined, because he bellowed like a baited bull, grabbed my upper arms, and squeezed. I couldn't break free. Without thinking, I stretched up and kissed him on a greasy cheek.

He backed away as if I had hit him with a fence post, his mouth agape. He didn't know whether to spit or cry. Nothing is more powerful than a kiss, especially with his kind.

He lurched toward the open doorway. Then we heard horses come stomping and snorting into the yard. Men shouted. Herman stepped back inside. I dug out my pistol and walked over to the doorway and looked out just as the sun was about to set. It was early for nightriders.

All but one of the six men were local. They lolled in their saddles while Irmgard Trefmann stood solid as a boulder, with one hand on her little girl's shoulder, the other in her apron pocket.

Mace Brown got off his white-legged sorrel. He fiddled for most of our socials, though he wasn't much good. "Where's your old man and Herman?" he asked Irmgard in slurred words. "We want to talk to them."

"They go to Topeka for safety," she answered.

Mace and one of the other farmers, both unsteady on their feet, pushed by her with their rifles held ready and entered her cabin. Irmgard waited outside, abusing the men on horseback with harsh-sounding German insults.

Mac tromped back onto the porch. "They ain't there."

Irmgard seemed ready to cry. Then everyone looked over at me.

"Katherine Ann, what are you doing out here?" Mace asked me.

"Boarding," I replied.

"With *abolitionists?*" he sputtered.

Herman and his pa were abolitionists, not Irmgard. She was just a wife with a fool husband. She had flailed at locusts, beat out prairie fires, birthed children alone, lost two of them, and endured both blizzards and drought and probably a few beatings from her husband. Herman was worth saving just because of her.

"That's the agreement," I said.

Mace walked toward me. His breath would have pickled an egg.

"You ain't coming in here, Mace Brown," I told him.

He laughed. I cocked my Colt and pointed it at his chest.

"Katie, you wouldn't kill anybody," he said.

"You're right." I swung my aim at his horse. "But I'll ruin your horse."

He snickered. "You sure you can hit it?"

"I can knock a tick off it from here," I said.

He cursed. "You shoot my horse, Little Miss, and I'll break your arm."

"You touch me, Mace Brown, and my pa will butcher you like a pig," I threatened.

One of the farmers chuckled. "She's got you there, Mace. Her pa was whelped by a she-wolf."

"I ain't scared of him," Mace muttered. But he stayed rock still. "They anybody in there, Katherine Ann?" gesturing at the sod hut.

I answered his question with a question so I wouldn't have to lie, "What would a man be doing in my soddy?"

Mace went pale like he had just seen a ghost, probably his own if my pa ever thought he questioned my virtue.

"I didn't mean nothing like that, Katie Ann, and *you* know it." He stood there a moment, then mounted and rode off with the pack of drunks following him.

Herman came out. "I don't owe you nothing," he told me

234

right off. "I could of took care of them myself." He stomped off toward the cabin.

Irmgard shooed her other two children in after him. She then came over to me shy as a dove. Her breath caught on a sob. "I cannot say enough thanks." And when she hugged me, I felt the hardness of a pistol in her apron pocket.

The August of Still Another Year

by

Carolyn Banks

The hounds combing the hillside woke me up this morning. I tried to block their voices out, but they called to each other at odd intervals, making that impossible.

I went outside to feed the chickens, fearing, I couldn't tell you why, the rushing sound their wings would make while they flapped over to take up what I'd tossed them. Grain. Rat dung scattered through it. I never knew how the rats could do it, penetrate the tight-lidded cans.

The cat was nowhere to be found. Flattened under the shed, probably, because of those hounds.

A pickup truck came down the road, a boy who looked too young to drive at the wheel. And a girl who bounced as a doll might, stiff and loose at the same time, too close beside him. The truck was far off, but I could see, all the same, the bright red rouge spots on the girl's cheeks. Big as fifty-cent pieces, and just as round.

I turned away. Stared out at the dusty dry fields. The sun was already too hot. The creek bed was chapped and looked as though it always had been. I brought water by hand to the pony, losing most of it along the way.

236

I called my son in Denver, told him something was wrong. I'm afraid, I said.

You're always afraid, he reminded me.

I heard his wife say, Is that your mother again?

The flapping sound, more of it. He is shushing her, waving, I suppose, their bedsheets.

What time is it out there? I ask him.

Early, he says, I told you before how to figure that out.

I walk out onto the porch and think about the hounds, wondering when it was their calling to each other stopped. It is too early by a week or more to be running hounds.

It is always too something, I recognize.

I make my way to the line and take the towels down. They are sooty, but I fold them the same as if they weren't. Then the cat comes by at last, wanting cottage cheese. I go inside to oblige. I feed him right up on the table. After he eats, he makes a bed out of the towels. I am regaining something when the telephone interrupts it.

Mom, he says.

I thought you'd be at work by now, I tell him.

I am at work, he says.

He has the kind of job where he can make a call to Virginia and not get into trouble for it.

We were thinking, Mom, that we'd fly back home to see you.

Oh, I say, sarcastic-like. So it's that time.

He never hears. He doesn't try. He tells me, There's a flight in the morning. We can rent a car at the airport. How does that sound?

Like a rush of feathers at my ankles, that's how. Like cold grey wings. Like seeing Sally with her rouge spots, sitting way too close the way she'd do the minute she thought the car was far enough down the lane.

You don't have to come, I say, and I hear him let his breath out like he's been holding it in.

You're sure? he asks me.

I don't even have to weigh it anymore, the flapping that I fear against the rest. I'm sure, I say, holding him and what is certainly the end—my end—at bay.

237

Fine China and
Feathered Friends

by

Charlotte L. Babcock

Aunt Em was especially proud of her dining room. It was without question the brightest room in her small house. Large double windows on two adjoining walls allowed sunlight to reflect off the fancy dishes displayed on plate rails along the inner walls. The reflected light made shimmery images as it danced across her highly polished Queen Anne dining set. Pampered house plants on shelves beneath the windows provided a year-round balance of greenery and wonderful blossoms. Aunt Em had a way with plants, and with birds, too, as Uncle Ted discovered.

Uncle Ted liked peace and quiet, particularly at mealtime. "Live and let live," he'd say when Aunt Em would remark about the behavior of certain relatives. "If it doesn't hurt us, it's not our concern." He was patient with children and he thought animals should run free. "Live and let live doesn't mean tying them up or putting them in a cage," he'd explain to any youngster who wanted to keep a found turtle or baby bird. "Wild animals are meant to be free."

His patience, however, was put to a double test when Aunt Em, who had wanted a bird for years, brought home a canary, put it in the dining room, and declared firmly that it was there to stay.

The bird cage hung on a stand between the windows. The canary, an expensive and wonderful singer, would puff out its throat and fill the whole house with song whenever household noises—the hum of the vacuum or the rattling of dishes—inspired it to sing. The greater the commotion, the louder the canary sang. At mealtime its song was loud enough to interfere with normal conversation, and that is what led to the bird's undoing.

Uncle Ted did not appreciate a caged and noisy bird disrupting his meals, but after fifty years with Aunt Em he knew better than to complain, so for most of the spring he suffered quietly through this mealtime disturbance. He did, however, devise a technique to shut the bird up.

Whenever the canary would burst forth, Uncle Ted would suddenly wave his arm in the air. The motion would startle the canary into a few moments of silence. At the start of the next song, Uncle Ted would wave again. And so it would go until Uncle Ted left the table.

Uncle Ted's suffering changed form on Father's Day. Aunt Em had invited the whole family and was busy cleaning and baking for days ahead. She added leaves to the table and set out her best china and silver. She was so busy that she didn't miss the canary until one of the children asked about it. Puzzled, Aunt Em stared at the empty cage for an instant. Then she shot a murderous look at Uncle Ted who shrugged but said nothing. A few days later, after a neighbor reported seeing a bright yellow bird in her lilac bush, Aunt Em stopped speaking to Uncle Ted.

Aunt Em stubbornly left the empty cage in the dining room and took to eating alone in the kitchen while Uncle Ted found excuses to eat in town. Whenever anyone asked about the situation Uncle Ted would politely change the subject. Aunt Em refused to comment at all.

In mid-July there was another family occasion for Aunt Em to celebrate and she made her usual preparations. When she went to set the table, Aunt Em found a blue parakeet preening its feathers in the canary cage. Attached to the cage was a tag on which the question "Truce?" was scrawled.

Unlike the canary, the parakeet found no inspiration in

mealtime sounds and it went unnoticed by the others until it happened to squawk as dessert was being served. Aunt Em explained the bird's presence with terse honesty. "I've been wanting a bird since Father's Day. Now I have one." She placed a piece of raspberry pie on a plate and extended it across the table to Uncle Ted. "Your favorite," she said sweetly. Uncle Ted showed visible relief as he gratefully nodded his thanks.

Soon Em and Ted were again eating together in the dining room. By fall it appeared that everyone had forgotten about the canary. The parakeet would squawk occasionally at mealtimes but Uncle Ted didn't seem to mind. He was, in fact, pleased that every morning Aunt Em would take the bird out of its cage to ride on her shoulder as she went about her housework. She talked to it and fed it treats while Uncle Ted privately congratulated himself for having made peace.

But all this time Aunt Em was working on revenge.

It came about on Thanksgiving. The family was seated, heads bowed, waiting for Uncle Ted to say grace when a voice from the bird cage unmistakably intoned, "Bad boy, bad boy, Ted." Two of the younger grandchildren began to giggle and Aunt Em quickly shushed them with a stern look. She tried to pretend she hadn't heard the parakeet, but the smug expression on her face gave her away. All the while they'd been doing the housework together, Em had been teaching the bird to talk. Now she was pleased with the results.

"Bad boy," the bird repeated again. This time adult snickering joined the children's. Aunt Em smiled. Then she put her finger to her lips. "Ssssh," she whispered. "It's time for Grace."

Uncle Ted, head still bowed, knew all eyes were on him and he blushed brightly before he started to pray. "Thank you for all that's before us, Lord," he said reverently. Then, raising his head, he looked straight at Aunt Em and softly added, "especially those who can teach birds to talk."

Moving North

by

Barbara Lau

He warned me:
    you do not truly know something
    until you have eaten it.

I stuffed the car with ice scrapers, wool socks
and antifreeze. But I still did not believe:
    that one gray cloud squatting over the city
    could hatch winter,
    that the sun could burn on so short a wick,
    or that geese could shake the trees bare
    as they flew overhead.

Now sleet blanches the city.
Cars go lame.
Sidewalks trip me up.
I eat gallons of snow cream
and try to grasp the world
in black and white.

Angie

by

Patricia Garfinkel

Angie holds her eyes closed against the morning sunlight that
dances with the blowing snow outside her bedroom window.
Holding on to her own warmth under the covers, she wonders
why she is still in bed. She was never one to lie around in the
morning. An inner spring always seemed to push her out of bed
even on Sunday mornings when the store was closed and Frankie
didn't have to get up. Even when she didn't feel well she'd force
herself out of bed to take a hot shower. There was something
safer in being up and about.

She remembers being a child afraid of staying home from
school. Lying in bed in the quiet apartment opened the doors of
fantasy and brought a fear that broke her will to move.

"Not feeling well, my Angie?" her mother would ask. "You
won't miss much in a day. I'll ask Marie to bring your work home.
In the refrigerator there's leftover minestrone for lunch. We'll
talk a little later."

Her mother would lean over the bed; the smell of mothballs
hung in her wool robe. With one hand she pulled the satin com-
forter up around Angie's shoulders. The coarse skin on her fingers snagged along the glossy fabric. Angie gritted her teeth

242

against the sound. The other hand came down like a verdict on Angie's forehead.

Watching her mother's ample breasts tilt toward her face, Angie already knew the words. "Almost a hundred. I told you not to go out without your umbrella the other day. You know you always catch a cold from wet hair."

After so many days of her childhood spent trapped in the cramped apartment filled with ornate furniture, Angie developed a busy briskness about herself. When her children were young, she'd be dressed and in the kitchen before they'd shuffle out of their rooms in their flannel sleepers. Already she would have seen Frankie off to the shop after preparing fried eggs and ham, half a grapefruit, and two cups of black coffee. He had eaten the same breakfast since the day they were married.

This morning in bed, time closes in on her like an accordion. The Italian section of Philadelphia where she grew up bustles behind her closed eyes. How many years ago was it that she first caught Frankie looking at her in English class? Everything happened so predictably from then on. They dated, went steady, went to the Senior Prom and were married by Father Valenza a year later.

In the beginning, they struggled side by side. Two boys, two years apart, and Frankie making a go of the radio-TV repair shop, coming home every day for lunch until they got a small house in the suburbs. Then it was too far to come home and Angie packed salami on Italian bread with lots of mustard, a package of Hostess cupcakes and some potato chips. Every day the same breakfast, every day the same lunch.

Sometimes she'd ask, "Frankie, don't you ever want to try something different?"

His answer was always the same. "When a man likes the way it is, no reason to part his hair a different way." He never even liked it when she would change the furniture around in the living room. And once she went out and got her hair cut short in the latest style; Frankie was furious. He said she didn't look like the girl

243

he married anymore. He got even madder when her mother said to him, "Whose hair do you think it is anyway?"

He snapped back, "She's my wife and I'll tell her the way I like it. Anyway, I bring home the bacon here and enough of it, too."

She recalls being in bed that night as if it were yesterday. As Frankie tossed restlessly on his side of the bed and moved his pillow to create a wall between them, she thought back to her schooldays and how she and Marie would talk about what kind of man they each would marry. Marie used to say that Angie's long hair could catch anyone. Angie thought that Marie's thick ankles and waist and her bushy eyebrows would make it hard for her. She was pleased by her own good looks and enjoyed the lack of competition from her best friend.

Funny how things turned out. Marie went to secretarial school and got a job at an insurance company. That's where she met Eddie, one of the salesmen. He was eight years older and had been overseas during the war. He liked to travel and each year they took their two weeks of vacation in a different place. One year they went to Canada and Marie brought Angie one of those fancy tortoise-shell combs. Angie remembered swirling her hair to one side and fastening it with the comb for Marie to see. She snapped her fingers like castanets and shouted, "Olé!" They both laughed, but it hurt Angie to hear about the exotic places that Marie and Eddie had been to and that she had only heard about. Frankie's idea of a vacation was a weekend in the Poconos with his parents and brother and sister-in-law and their kids.

She rolls over in bed and opens her eyes to face the pillow. Out of the corner of her eye she catches sight of a ringlet of her long hair against the rumpled pillow slip. It seems almost as if the hair belongs to someone else and she is a stranger noticing it from a distance. She's surprised at the number of gray hairs among the dark brown. She reaches out and holds the ringlet in her fingers. The gray hairs are coarser and more unruly than the others. Somehow the rich brown sensuality of her hair seems to have suddenly disappeared.

Frankie used to run his fingers through her long hair, making the music of her body ripple out to him like a strummed harp. It was always her hair that turned Frankie on. Maybe that's why he got so upset the time she cut it. He would say, "Let's go to bed and do God's work." In bed he would always touch her hair first as if it were the switch that turned the power on. One night when he said the same thing about God's work, she remembers thinking how she wished he could find some other way to say it: maybe "I'm gonna take that long dark hair to bed and you can come, too."

For a moment a mixture of anger and regret floods over Angie as she realizes that Frankie is the only man who ever touched her that way—ever touched her body that way. Somewhere the excitement and electricity between them had vanished. She hadn't really noticed it until about a year after her operation. It seemed so long ago. Two years after Tony was born she had the first miscarriage. She was three months pregnant and started spotting. Doc Rizzo ordered her to bed, but Frankie Junior and Tony were just tots then and she couldn't stay in bed. She didn't want to anyway.

That first morning when she tried, she felt a panic rush through her body like the feeling she had had when she was trapped in the elevator at Wanamaker's department store. When the panic hit and nausea made her whole body break out in a cold sweat, she sat bolt upright in bed hoping not to vomit. When the wave subsided, she lay back on the pillows, her blue nylon nightgown wet and cold against her body. Grabbing her damp hair in both hands, she covered her face. "Oh, God, get me out of bed," she cried. Frankie Junior was hovering at the side of the bed asking, "Why is Mommy crying?" She pulled him up onto the bed next to her, the miniature wooden soldier clutched in his hand digging into the side of her neck. Her hair cascaded over his tiny shoulders like a cape. Three days later the baby was gone.

The time between when she lost the first baby and the second is a blur to her now. The only vivid memory is Christmas Eve dinner at Frankie's mom's house. They were all seated around the heavy mahogany table, fifteen of them, when Frankie's dad raised his glass and toasted, "To Frankie and Angie and lots more grandbabies." Angie blushed right to the center of her being.

Frankie's retort still rang in her ears. "Don't worry, Papa, she won't lose a baby again, eh, Angie?" And he tugged on her hair that was almost shoulder length again, but not long enough for him yet. He leaned over and whispered in her ear, "Soon your hair will be long enough to have another baby."

She remembers lying awake that night wondering why Frankie didn't remember that she hadn't cut her hair until after she lost the baby. She had never challenged him on it. Somehow she knew he needed to think of it that way.

After she lost the second baby, Doc Rizzo said she would have to have the operation. The night she told Frankie what Doc said, he left and didn't come home till very late. He said something about needing to go over the shop's inventory.

The surgery left Angie weak for a long time. For the first few weeks her mother stayed with them. She wanted Angie to rest in bed. Each time Angie tried, she felt like she was being smothered by the pillows and comforters. She would hear the late bell for school ringing in her ears. Late for what? Where was she supposed to be?

At night she and Frankie would lie in bed not even touching. After the last check-up, Doc Rizzo said they could resume normal relations. Frankie said he was still worried and wanted to wait longer. On the night they made love for the first time since the surgery, Frankie was reluctant. Angie thought it was Frankie's fear of hurting her and she tried to gently reassure him.

Months passed and Frankie seemed to be so distant, as if a glass jar had been pulled down over him. Angie could see him perfectly, but he was unreachable. One night she had a dream that her head was tucked in the crook of the elbow of a dark and handsome guitarist; her hair was stretched out along the length of the guitar strings and the guitarist was strumming a wild Mexican song.

She woke from the dream wanting Frankie to hold her. He was in a dead sleep over on the edge of his side of the bed. Angie remembered that ever since the operation Frankie had not talked about God's work. She wanted to ask him why and had formed the question in a thousand different ways.

One evening when it was just the two of them for dinner, Angie poured wine and lit the blue candles in her grandmother's candlesticks. Some time after her second glass of wine she felt the tense space between her and Frankie mellow a bit, or was it the tenseness within her about Frankie, or was it Frankie looking softer in the candlelight? She swirled the wine in her glass for a moment, holding the glass stem between her thumb and forefinger. Then raising her glass a little bit too high for a proper toast, she said, "To God and his work! He's been unemployed too long, don't you think, Frankie?"

"Stop talking nonsense, Angie. You've had too much wine." He pushed his chair back to leave the table and then leaned forward toward her. "Where'd you get that silly comb in your hair?" His rough fingers plucked it out as if it were a bird feather. Angie's hair fell forward, partially covering her face and the tears that began to pool in her eyes.

The sharp sunlight filling the room this morning finally forces Angie out of her reverie. She looks at the clock and realizes that she only has an hour to shower, dress, and drive to the beauty shop for the noon haircut appointment she made two weeks ago. She closes her eyes again and can see the clumps of her thick hair falling one by one to the floor until a horseshoe of hair surrounds the beautician's chair. What is it they say about horseshoes? If you hold them upside down, your luck runs out. Looking over at her hair again on the pillow slip, her mind holds one ringlet apart, the one she wants to leave on Frankie's pillow tonight.

It'll Be All Right— Doncha Know

by

Tom Davis

Uncle Bud didn't move. The pool of blood he lay in grew larger with each heartbeat. He was naked except for a towel covering his feet. Aunt Josie couldn't do anything but hiccup and cry. Beau, thumping his tail nervously against the wall, hid under the sewing machine table. His big brown eyes darted between me, Aunt Josie, and Uncle Bud. It wasn't Beau's fault, but I was afraid I was the only one who'd see it that way.

It all happened when Mama had Marrlee, my sister, and appendicitis all at the same time. Aunt Josie was keeping me and Beau for a week or so until Mama was better.

I like staying with Aunt Josie and Uncle Bud, especially Uncle Bud. Even though Daddy can't stand being in the same room with him, of all my uncles, he's my favorite.

Uncle Bud cusses and tells dirty jokes around me. He even slips me a cigarette now and again and turns the other way while I sneak a swallow of his beer. Of course, all this happens when Aunt Josie's not around.

The day before the accident, Aunt Josie and I were at my house visiting Mama and the new baby. Everybody carried on like she was the prettiest baby ever. Actually, she looked like a big pink possum.

Everybody was complimenting Mama on how well she looked. I don't know why. She didn't look so good to me. Just then Aunt Lasa came in from Atlanta. Aunt Lasa never entered a room—she *burst* into it. And sure enough, things seemed brighter. Daddy used to say that she could find something good about an axe murder.

The first thing Aunt Lasa did was give me a big hug. Then she sat by Mama and started cheering her up, which was something I thought Mama needed at the time.

"Girl," said Aunt Lasa, patting Mama's hand, "it was just plain luck—doncha know? Here you check into the hospital to have a baby and get your appendix taken out at the same time. Why, just think of all the money you and Hoyt saved. And you were going to feel bad anyway, so why not get it all over with at one time—doncha know?"

And so it went until Aunt Lasa had everyone in the room convinced that Mama was the luckiest woman in the world and they'd saved enough money on operations to put us all through college.

It was time to go, so I went with Aunt Josie. Aunt Lasa was spending the night with Maw Maw and Paw Paw, so she went with them.

The accident happened the next morning.

I was staying in a guest bedroom that Aunt Josie had turned into a sewing room. I'd stuck my underwear and things in the middle drawer of this big oak dresser.

When I packed my stuff, I slipped Sneaky, a pet grass snake into my bag. Sneaky lived in a mayonnaise jar. I'd soaked its label off, punched holes in its top with an ice pick, and stuffed it half full of weeds.

When I unpacked, I hid Sneaky in a drawer near the top that didn't look used much.

That morning I was standing in my underwear, poking around in my drawer. I'd fished out a shirt and socks, and was

249

about to grab my shorts, when Aunt Josie came in. "Excuse me Rip, I need my spare pair of glasses."

I stepped back. Aunt Josie opened Sneaky's drawer and found the mayonnaise jar.

"What in the world?" Aunt Josie couldn't see so well without her glasses. And before I could warn her, she had Sneaky's jar against her nose.

Sneaky poked his head up to the glass and stuck out his tongue. I can still hear the scream Aunt Josie let out. She went one way; Sneak's jar went the other, crashing into the wall above the dresser. Everything, including Sneaky, fell behind it.

The door flew open and there stood Uncle Bud. His hair—what little he had—was matted and parted on either side of his ears. A red, white, and blue striped beach towel stretched tight around his considerable middle. A stubby cigar was wedged into the corner of his mouth. "Josie, what in God's name is going on?" Uncle Bud asked, his big face reflecting the moment's excitement.

"Snake!" blurted Aunt Josie, pointing toward the dresser.

"Don't anybody move," Uncle Bud commanded and tore from the room.

Aunt Josie wasn't about to stand near that dresser, so she ran over to Beau and me and hugged me around the shoulders.

I opened my mouth to explain that it was just a harmless grass snake when Uncle Bud appeared in the doorway, coat hanger in one hand and nickel-plated pistol in the other.

"Bud! What do you think you're doing with that gun?" Aunt Josie asked, squeezing my shoulders so tight I thought I'd lose my breath.

"Stay back, Josie. I know what I'm doing. Leave me alone." Uncle Bud got down on all fours and started scratching the coat hanger under the dresser.

I've come to reason that when somebody, especially an adult, declares he knows what he's doing and says to leave him alone that he usually doesn't, but you'd better.

While Uncle Bud was crawling around the floor, the towel worked itself loose. Beau, naturally curious, walked over and sniffed Uncle Bud's bottom. Unfortunately, he got too close.

The next thing I know, Uncle Bud lets out a holler and raises straight up crashing his head into the drawer I'd left open. The pistol went off, rattling the windows.

When the smoke cleared, Uncle Bud had knocked himself out and in the process shot off his middle finger and meanwhile Aunt Josie was crying and calling for the Lord's help. Beau was hiding under the table, Uncle Bud was lying there bleeding all over the floor, and I was 'bout to wet my pants.

Aunt Josie finally pulled herself together enough to call the hospital. She told me to wait outside and bring 'em in. She wasn't about to leave Uncle Bud.

Hardly five minutes later, the ambulance fishtailed around the corner. Eugene Butterbottom and Mike Cavanaugh got out and ran up carrying a stretcher. Eugene was tall and skinny with the head of a chicken. Mike was average height and a little potbellied. His long brown hair was pulled into a pony tail and he smiled a lot for no good reason.

I showed 'em where Uncle Bud was. The first words out of Eugene's mouth were, "God-all-mighty, he's bleeding like a stuck pig!" Eugene wasn't known for his bedside manner.

"Look-a-here what I found," said Mike, holding up Uncle Bud's finger and beaming his crooked smile.

"Gimme that." Eugene dug out a handkerchief from his back pocket. "Sometimes they can sew 'em back on."

Eugene and Mike fiddled with Uncle Bud while Aunt Josie and I watched helplessly. After they'd stopped the bleeding, they wrestled his 300 pounds to a belly-up position on the stretcher. The robe Aunt Josie had thrown over him fell off and he was showing himself again.

"Rip, get the front door," Aunt Josie said. "I'm calling your Daddy. Be there directly."

I opened the door and followed Eugene and Mike out. Both cussed as they struggled with Uncle Bud.

Eugene was leading when he stumbled. Mike and I watched as Uncle Bud, stretcher, and Eugene tumbled down the front steps. This was not Uncle Bud's day. They gathered him back up on the stretcher.

Eugene said, "Rip, if you won't say anything and the doctor can't sew that finger back on, I'll make sure you get it."

Before I could answer, Aunt Josie ran up, and off they went, siren blasting.

I sat on the front porch hugging my knees, thinking about the finger and about what I would tell Daddy. I worried about Beau. I remembered when Jimmy Burton's dog wouldn't stop chasing old man Kendrick's goats, Jimmy had to give him away. I reckoned that what had happened to Uncle Bud on account of Beau was worse than chasing goats. Daddy was never too thrilled about the way Beau chewed up things. On occasions he even referred to him as that "good-for-nothing dog."

On the way to the hospital I told Daddy everything that had happened—except the part about Eugene and Mike dropping Uncle Bud. For Beau's sake I tried not to make it sound so bad. It had started with Sneaky, after all.

Daddy and I walked into the waiting room. Aunt Josie was perched on a green Naugahyde sofa turning the pages of a *Saturday Evening Post* but not really seeing 'em.

"How's he doing Josie?" Daddy usually referred to Uncle Bud as "that no-account-Bud," but when Daddy was around Aunt Josie he always called him "he" or "your husband."

"Doctor Malloy says he'll be okay, Hoyt," she said.

I thought I saw disappointment on Daddy's face.

We heard the door open behind us and Aunt Lasa burst into the room. "Josie," she said running over and giving Aunt Josie a one-armed hug, "everything's going to be all right—doncha know? Why, while Bud's laid up here, I bet he'll lose fifty pounds. And the best thing to take your mind off this is to go shopping. We'll pry some money out of Paw Paw and buy that sofa you've been talking about—doncha know?"

Aunt Josie was in good hands, so Daddy turned me around and we left to pick up Beau and my stuff.

I said nothing until we pulled into the driveway. "Daddy, what are you going to do about Beau?"

Daddy thought a minute, cleared his throat, looked at me, and, as a big smile stretched across his face, said, "One thing I'm *not* going to do. I'm not ever going to call Beau a 'good-for-nothing dog' again."

From that day on Daddy and Beau were best friends. I never did tell anybody about Eugene and Mike dropping Uncle Bud, even when they were trying to figure out how his wrist got broken.

And Eugene was as good as his word. I've got the finger in a little bottle of formaldehyde hid under the house. Mike offered me five dollars for it, but I'm gonna hang onto it a while longer.

Aunt Lasa's right. It's a mighty bad bundle that doesn't have a little good stuffed into it somewhere—doncha know?

Starry, Starry Night

by

Jan Bowman

"What are we looking at, Daddy?" the children ask.

"The sky," he answers. "Starry, starry nights." His sleepy-eyed children stand shivering, teeth chattering from excitement and the cool air. Ice crystals form tents on the brown autumn lawn.

"Maybe we'll see a meteor shower," he says. Bending down, he wraps a blanket around his youngest daughter. He smooths her blonde straight hair and tucks the blanket under her chin. His shoes make crunching noises on the stiff frozen stalks of grass.

"Or maybe," he says, straightening up slowly, "the sky has a surprise for us tonight." He looks up at the sky and turns to examine the moon, stroking his jaw with a strong square hand.

On clear, cold nights he awakens his children—two girls and a boy. He wraps them in soft flannel blankets and takes them outside to watch the heavens with him. Breathing deeply, he makes their breath visible by warming it in his cheeks and letting it out in controlled explosions. It amuses his children. His brown eyes soften at the sounds of their laughter. "Music," he says and he smiles at their pleasure.

Wearing a blue woolen shirt and, if it is windy, hands in his pockets, he whistles a tuneless song about the sky. "Watch over there," he says pointing toward the moon.

254

"Look!" The oldest girl shouts and points toward the western sky. Her dark curly head bobs as she jumps up and down.

"Shooting stars! Look, Daddy," shrieks the younger girl. Her blonde head pops out of the blanket. "Oh, they're beautiful."

"Comets," says the older sister. "They're comets. Dozens of them. Like sparklers. Look! Quick!"

"Where?" screams the boy. "Can't see. Show me."

"Wow! A meteor shower. Look at them go." The man picks up his son and holds him high in the air, braced against his shoulder. The boy is the baby, only three. The man points. "Look, do you see them now?" he asks. The sparkling lights flash across the sky, glitter for a few moments, and sink into the horizon.

"Can we make a wish, Daddy?" asks the blonde girl. Her blanket falls away from her shoulders and trails behind her. "Can we?"

"Are shooting stars and meteors the same thing?" the oldest girl asks. "Can we make one wish or…"

"Or can we make lots of wishes, since we saw lots of stars?" interrupts the younger girl. She tugs on the blanket and turns in circles to wrap it around her shoulders.

"Sure, you can make as many wishes as you need," their father says.

"We all got to see this one, Daddy," says the oldest girl. "Except Mommy missed it again."

"I wish Mommy would look at the sky with us," says the younger girl. She sniffs and wipes her cold nose on the blanket.

"I wish Mommy would feel better," says the older girl. She pulls her blanket around her like a small, blue tepee. Her teeth chatter in the cold air.

"I wish that too," says the man. His brown eyes glisten. "Don't yell too loud. You'll wake her up." He kneels on the ground beside the girls. The boy remains in his arms and he shifts the boy onto his shoulders. He gathers a daughter under each arm. They brace themselves against his strength. Knowing he is solid, they lean against him and they are warmed.

"Why are we still looking at the sky, Daddy?" asks the oldest of the girls. She wipes her eyes and yawns.

"Why?" the boy chirps as he snuggles against the man's

rough evening beard. The boy pats his father's face and rubs his chubby baby fingers along the bristles of the man's dark stubble.

"Because we're going to see an eclipse," the man says, and he breathes in the cold air and takes satisfaction in the freshly bathed, sweet smells of his children. "Because the sky seems the same, but it's always changing."

"The moon's always changing," says the younger girl and she twists the button on the sleeve of the man's woolen shirt. "Sometimes it's round and sometimes it's just a little sliver." Her soft face is framed by the satin binding around the edge of the blanket.

"What is it, Daddy?" asks the boy sleepily.

"Eclipse," says the older girl. "Daddy just told you."

"What?" asks the boy again and he rubs his eyes with his fist. He drapes his arms around the man's head.

"Eclipse makes the night special." The man pauses, "Every night is special. But we'll never see the sky exactly like it looks tonight. The sky, like everything, changes."

"But why?" asks the boy from his position sitting on the man's broad shoulders. He curls the man's thick hair around the fingers on one hand and secretly sucks his thumb on his other.

The man points to the sky and gently, one by one, takes each child's fingers and points them toward the full harvest moon. "Look," he says, "the eclipse is beginning." Clouds clear away. A shadow covers the cool blonde moon like a soft flannel blanket. The moon disappears for a time and reappears as a large black oval, like a face wrapped in a shroud and encircled with white satin bindings of light.

"Look," says the oldest girl. "The moon has a ring of light around it. Looks like it's wearing a hat made out of light."

"Corona," says the man softly. "The ring of light is called a corona."

"Cromma," says the boy. He pats his father's head and leans sleepily against his neck.

256

The children watch silently as the moon returns to normal. The only sound they hear is their father's watch ticking next to their ears.

"This eclipse is special," he says. "You and I will be gone the next time the moon and the sun line up this way again."

Notes on Contributors

JEAN ADAIR is an award-winning fiction writer who lives in Melrose, Minnesota. She also writes nonfiction, poetry, gags for cartoonists and career profiles for Vocational Biographies of Sauk Centre.

JIM ADAMS' stories have appeared in many books, newspapers and magazines. His story, "Goodbye Venice," originally appeared in *Il Caffe*. He lives on a tree ranch in Washington state, south of Mount St. Helens.

CHARLOTTE L. BABCOCK is a former junior high school English teacher who lives and writes in central Vermont. She has been a contributor to several national magazines, including *Country Woman*. Her stories and essays appear frequently in a variety of local publications.

KRISTINA D. BAGULEY, who lives in Houston, Texas, is an aerospace engineer and a pilot. In her spare time, she enjoys writing about people and has had many of her stories published.

CAROLYN BANKS, co-editor of both volumes of *A Loving Voice*, has recently had four novels published and is currently authoring a mystery series set in the equestrian world. The first of these, *Death by Dressage*, was just published by Fawcett. She lives in Elgin, Texas.

JUDITH BELL's novel, *Real Love*, won the 1989 Washington Prize for fiction. Her short stories have appeared in a number of prestigious magazines, including *Short Fiction by Women*. An art historian in Arlington, Virginia, she writes about the arts for magazines including *Art and Antiques*, *Elle* and *Omni*, among others.

SALLY BELLEROSE, a nurse as well as a writer, has had her work appear in numerous publications, including *Sojourner, Word of Mouth, Women's Glibber* and *Caprice*. She presently lives in Northampton, Massachusetts.

LUCILLE BELLUCCI has had many works of fiction for both children and adults published. These include essays, poetry, humor, satire and features. Born in Shanghai, she now resides in Oakland, California. Currently, she has three novels making the rounds.

JAN BOWMAN lives in Columbia, Maryland, where she is working on two collections of short stories. She's an educator at the Montgomery County Public Schools and occasionally acts as a consultant to the Department of Education.

JACK BOYD's story, "Of Gophers and Boys at New Year's," first appeared in the *Abilene Reporter-News*. He has had several books on music published, including a college text entitled *Encore!* He has also published books on religion, among them, *One God, One Child*. He lives in Abilene, Texas.

JOHN BUCHHOLZ was raised in New York's idyllic Finger Lakes region and much of his writing reflects his childhood experiences there. His stories have appeared in numerous magazines, including *Byline*. He's also had nonfiction work published in *Mr. Guitar* and *Down Memory Lane*. He lives in Paoli, Pennsylvania.

ERIK BUNDY has lived and worked overseas for the past eleven years. Currently he lives in a castle in Limburg, a southern province of The Netherlands. His stories and poems have appeared in many literary magazines.

J. JORDAN CANNADY is an editorial cartoonist and columnist with over 200 cartoons and 70 columns published in various newspapers. His short stories have appeared in *Concho River Review, Byline* and *Transitions*, among others. He is slated to appear in the forthcoming *King Magician Warrior Weenie*, an anthology of humor that deals with the men's movement. He lives in Stephenville, Texas.

NANCY CLIMER's first published story appeared in the first volume of *A Loving Voice*. She is a homemaker married to a retired Army officer. She lives in Las Vegas, Nevada.

MARY CONNORS describes herself as a "part-time respiratory therapist, part-time student, part-time writer and full-time bargain hunter." She has won several writing contests and has a story scheduled for publication in the national magazine, *Women's World*. She lives in Ozark, Missouri.

E. SHAN CORREA lives in Hahaione Valley, Honolulu, where she is a full-time writer and editor of the *Japan-America Journal*. Her fiction, nonfiction and poetry have appeared in major regional and national publications.

TOM DAVIS is a career Special Forces Army colonel (Green Beret). He is the author of *What Would You Like on Your Mashed Potatoes?* — a collection of stories that chronicle the antics of a boy growing up in the rural South. He lives in Fayetteville, North Carolina and is presently writing an action adventure novel.

MICHAEL DIRDA, writer and editor for *The Washington Post Book World*, received the 1993 Pulitzer Prize in criticism for his essays and reviews. He currently lives in Silver Spring, Maryland.

CHUCK ETHERIDGE has been published in such literary journals as *Mesquite* and *Concho River Review*. His national publications are on what he terms "scholarly topics." He teaches at McMurry University and lives in Abilene, Texas.

FRANK FINALE, a teacher, has many published stories and poems to his credit. He is a founding member of the Ocean County Poets' Collective, which both he and his wife run. He lives in New Jersey.

LISA MARKS FISHER, a mother of three, was a contributing author to the first volume of *A Loving Voice*. She lives in Lake Forest, Illinois and is currently working on a novel.

JEAN FLYNN has spent 30 years in public education, 15 of them as a librarian. She is very busy with the lecture series that she gives, is active in school author visits, and also conducts workshops for teachers and librarians. She is married to Robert Flynn and lives in San Antonio, Texas.

ROBERT FLYNN is novelist-in-residence at Trinity University in San Antonio. Robert has authored four novels and has won numerous national awards.

DON GARDNER retired from the Coast Guard in 1970 and returned, "in spite of Thomas Wolfe's declaration," to his native North Carolina. In addition to writing, Don enjoys reading histories and biographies.

PATRICIA GARFINKEL has published two books of poetry, one of which won a competition for Washington-area writers. She works as a speechwriter in the U.S. House of Representatives and lives in Reston, Virginia.

BETTY GRAY's work appeared in the first volume of *A Loving Voice*. She recently completed a series of "nostalgia columns" for *The Westlake Picayune*, a newspaper published near her home in Bastrop, Texas.

LEE HILL-NELSON became a writer after she responded to a writing course advertisement in *Modern Maturity*. Her story that appears in this book, "Surviving with Sorghum," was first published in *Nostalgia* Magazine. She is a retired church secretary who lives in Waco, Texas. During World War II she served in the WAVES.

KATHLEEN HOFFMAN spent 25 years with community newspapers in her native Reva, Virginia, writing "about politics and unusual people, tragedies and oddball happenings, cars and animals." Her work appeared in the first volume of *A Loving Voice*.

EVELYN G. KENNEY has written a cookbook and several culinary articles. She works as a technical secretary in the Civil Engineering Department at Princeton University. Her interests include creating miniature Christmas trees for a local ballet production of *The Nutcracker*. She resides in Trenton, New Jersey.

CHERYL KERR's credits include national magazines and literary anthologies. She's also had a nonfiction book published and has completed a novel and a children's book. She is a CPA and college professor who lives in Austin, Texas.

JOHN H. LAMBE is a part-time writer who has a story included in the first volume of *A Loving Voice*. He enjoys writing about "the physically hard beauty of the West," among other things. He lives in Idabel, Oklahoma.

BARBARA LAU's poetry has appeared in numerous journals and anthologies, including *Spoon River Quarterly*, *A Loving Voice* and *When I Am an Old Woman I Shall Wear Purple*. She recently co-authored a nonfiction book entitled *You Don't Have to Go Home from Work Exhausted!* She lives in Austin, Texas.

MIKE LIPSTOCK, age 70, lives in Jericho, New York. He took up writing as a hobby three years ago. Since that time he has had over 50 stories published in a variety of magazines and his work has appeared in four anthologies. He is presently writing a screenplay.

BARBARA LUCEY writes that she "has spent much of her life either watching or making movies." She also tells us that among her heroes are "Colette, Jean Rhys, M.F.K. Fisher, Preston Sturges, George and Ira Gershwin, and Robert Parish — the oldest player in the NBA." This eclectic woman lives in Northampton, Massachusetts.

PAUL MILENSKI's story, "Walk," was first published in *Read Me*. Paul writes that he's sold hundreds of his stories and that many have been translated into other languages. Recently a prize-winning film was made that is based on his story "Tickits." He lives in Pittsfield, Massachusetts.

BETH S. MOORE's story that appears in this book, "The Longest Summer," reflects an incident from her childhood, which was spent in Lovell, Wyoming. Beth retired from teaching after 32 years and hopes to make writing a second career. She now lives in Hurricane, Utah.

KENNETH MORGAN has written a regular column for his local newspaper in Jasper, Texas for the past four years. His work will also soon appear in the *East Texas Historical Journal*. He has been a builder and a cabinet-maker for years.

IRL MOWERY studied meteorology, became an actor, a Broadway producer, and an opera company and ballet fundraiser. He has retired to write fiction, poetry and plays. He currently lives in Houston, Texas.

PHOEBE NEWMAN is a contributor to the first volume of *A Loving Voice*. She is in her fourth semester in the MFA Writing Program at Vermont College. She has had numerous poems and stories published in journals and anthologies. She lives in Los Alamos, New Mexico.

JANE HILL PURTLE lives in a log cabin in Bullard, Texas. She teaches English at local colleges, collects local histories and does editorial work when she's not writing. She's now working on an anthology of spiritual autobiographies of Southern women.

MARY CONNOR RALPH, whose work appeared in the first volume of *A Loving Voice*, is working on a collection of short stories illuminating the effect of landscape on people's lives. She lives in West Springfield, Massachusetts.

SUSAN RENSBERGER is a former White House speechwriter who is now working on a nonfiction book on child sexual abuse in the Mennonite community. She received a Reader's Choice award from *Prairie Schooner* for one of her short stories. She lives in Greenfield, Wisconsin.

INGRID RETI teaches creative writing and literature at California Polytechnic State University in San Luis Obispo where she also lives. She's a poet with two published collections entitled *Ephemera* and *Echoes of Silence*.

JANIS RIZZO is a licensed pharmacist, a former Air Force captain and a free-lance writer whose work has appeared in a number of national magazines. A mother of four young children, she is homeschooling the oldest two. Janis is co-editor of both *A Loving Voice* and *A Loving Voice II*. She lives in Cedar Creek, Texas.

MARJORIE ROMMEL teaches creative writing at Highline Community College and also runs a small public relations firm. Her poems, essays, stories, nonfiction and reviews have appeared in more than a hundred local, regional and national publications, including *The Observer* and *The Christian Science Monitor*. She lives in Auburn, Washington.

DOROTHY L. ROSE has had three collections of her poems published and her work has appeared in over 70 anthologies, magazines and journals. Born in Arkansas, she has lived in California since 1936.

LOIS SARGENT lives in Miami, Florida, where she is a psychologist who specializes in gestalt therapy, movement therapy and poetry therapy. She's won numerous awards for her poetry, which she says serves "as a bridge between my personal and professional life." Recently she taught English in Poland.

FLORA A. SCEARCE has won several awards for short stories, including one from the North Carolina Mothers' Association for "Quest for Nellie," which appears in this book. She belongs to an active writers' group and teaches Sunday School. She now lives in Havelock, North Carolina.

M.A. SCHAFFNER's poetry has appeared in numerous magazines, including *Negative Capability* and *Cumberland Poetry Review*. He recently had a short story published in *The Crescent Review*. He lives in Arlington, Virginia and works for the federal government in Washington, DC.

ELSIE SCHMIED's contribution to this book won a writing contest sponsored by a Knoxville newspaper. Elsie has also published numerous articles and book reviews. She worked 40 years as a nurse in the Midwest before retiring to Oakridge, Tennessee.

CLAUDIO G. SEGRÈ's short stories, personal essays, book reviews and columns have been published in national newspapers and magazines in the United States and in Italy. His most recent book is *Italo Balbo: A Fascist Life*. He has just completed a memoir about his father, Nobel Prize-winning physicist Emilio Segrè. He now lives in Austin, Texas.

SUSAN VOLCHOK has had short stories, articles, essays and a novella published. Her work has appeared in *Iris*, *The Virginia Quarterly* and *Paris Transcontinental*, among other literary journals. Her novella, *Sam's Girl*, was recently released on audiotape. She lives in New York City.

SONIA WALKER lives in Anchorage, Alaska where she attends the University of Alaska with the intention of eventually teaching elementary school. Her poetry has appeared in various journals, including *Writer's Companion* and *Omnific*.

ALLAN GEORGE WHITFIELD is completing his first novel, a techno-thriller. Born and raised in Brooklyn, New York, he now lives in Paoli, Pennsylvania. When not writing or playing basketball, Allan works actively in his own consulting firm.

CHRISTOPHER WOODS' story, "The Open House," which appears in this book, was originally published in *Story Time*. Christopher has had plays produced in New York, Chicago and Los Angeles and has also authored a novel entitled *The Dream Patch*. His stories have been widely published and he has been published in *Glimmer Train* and *Yankee*, among other journals. He now lives in Houston, Texas.

DOROTHY WINSLOW WRIGHT is a former Bostonian now living in Honolulu, Hawaii. She is an internationally published poet and writer whose work has appeared in *McCall's*, *Home Life*, *The Formalist* and *Manhattan Poetry Review*, among others. Her story, "A Sprig of Thyme," which appears in this book, was originally published in *The Herb Quarterly*.

Printed in the United States
203938BV00001B/292-363/A